Handbo
Practical Nursing

Handbook of
Practical Nursing

Margaret E. Crispin, SRN, BTA (Cert.), RNT

*Senior Nursing Officer, Teaching
Tutor-in-Charge, Pupil Nurse Training School,
The Princess Alexandra School of Nursing,
The London Hospital*

Foreword by Sheila M. Collins, OBE, BA, SRN, RSCN, RNT

*Director of Nursing Education,
(Tower Hamlets Health District),
The Princess Alexandra School of Nursing,
The London Hospital*

BAILLIÈRE TINDALL LONDON

A BAILLIÈRE TINDALL book published by
Cassell & Collier Macmillan Publishers Ltd
35 Red Lion Square, London WC1R 4SG
and at Sydney, Auckland, Toronto, Johannesburg
an affiliate of
Macmillan Publishing Co. Inc.
New York

First published as *Swire's Handbook for the Assistant Nurse* 1949
Sixth edition published as *Swire's Handbook of Practical Nursing* 1968
    Reprinted 1973
Handbook of Practical Nursing 1976

ISBN 0 7020 0557 6

Printed by William Clowes & Sons, Limited
London, Beccles and Colchester

Contents

Foreword by Sheila M. Collins, OBE, BA, SRN, RSCN, RNT

Preface

1.	The Human Life-Span	1
2.	Personal Health	5
3.	Aspects of Public Health	10
4.	Nutrition	13
5.	Household Pests and Parasites	20
6.	Accidents at home	24
7.	The Nurse in the Community by D. E. Brown, SRN, SCM, DTN, QN, RNT (Community), Senior Tutor, The Newham School of Community Nursing	28
8.	Mental Illness by R. B. Combes, SRN, RMN, RNT, Senior Tutor, The Princess Alexandra School of Nursing, The London Hospital	34
9.	The Nurse and the Hospital	51
10.	Care of the Patient in Bed	55
11.	Observing and Reporting	63
12.	Storage and Administration of Drugs	72
13.	The Surgical Patient	79
14.	Emergencies in the Ward	84
15.	Bandages, Splints and Slings	87
16.	Infection	93
17.	Nursing Care of the Young	105
18.	Nursing Care of the Elderly	113
19.	The Human Body	120
20.	Basic Physical Principles	125
21.	Bone	128
22.	Muscles and Joints	141
23.	The Respiratory System	146
24.	The Digestive System	151

25. Blood and Lymph   157
26. The Urinary Systems   170
27. The Reproductive Systems   179
28. The Skin   187
29. The Nervous System   202
30. The Special Senses   215
31. Hormones   224

Suggested Further Reading   230

Index   231

Foreword

This new edition of a practical nurse's textbook about nursing is particularly commendable. It is a guide, written by a skilful nurse, to the care of the patient—either at home or in hospital. It will be helpful to all entrants to basic nursing programmes. The simplicity of the text will be appreciated by nurses preparing for enrolment for whom it offers a comprehensive textbook. It should also encourage registered nurses and graduates to appreciate the need for firm foundations on which to build more advanced nursing studies. It is particularly appropriate that this revised edition should be published so soon after the recommendations of the Committee on Nursing have been accepted by the Secretary of State for Health and Social Services and when the integrated Health Service is becoming a reality.

February 1976   SHEILA M. COLLINS

Preface

This book has been written to introduce the basic aspects of nursing care to all those starting a career in nursing, a career which will take them into general and psychiatric hospitals, into peoples homes and into industry.

The advent of new drugs and treatments increases the responsibilities and the clinical importance of the nurse's role. Nurses are as a matter of course in close touch with their patients who are to them very real people and not merely cases; they are involved in the patient's recovery and rehabilitation though in many conditions the damage suffered is irreversible or there is a steady decline of physical function or mental acuity. Whatever the situation the nurse directs her efforts to the welfare of the patient.

The practical aspects of nursing care can be learnt only at the bedside but a sound foundation of knowledge is essential if the nurse is to carry out procedures with the confidence and manual skill which play so important a part in the patient's treatment.

The stresses of our world are themselves the cause of a great deal of illness; patients are subjected in addition, to tests, investigations and treatments which may embarrass, hurt or worry them. No-one will question the value of the advances made in science and medicine but what we must remember is that men and women have changed very little physically or emotionally over the years. Nurses still need the qualities of kindness, understanding and integrity and not always easy, a high degree of emotional stability.

Acknowledgements

I would like to thank my many nursing colleagues in the Princess Alexandra School of Nursing and in The London Hospital, for so generously giving their time for discussion of general principles of nursing and points of detail.

I would also like to thank Miss W. Huntly, SRN, SCM, RNT, DN (Lond.) for help and for typing the manuscript, Celia Perkins for preparing the illustrations and Mr T. R. Swinhoe of Baillière Tindall for encouragement and assistance with the text.

January 1976   MARGARET E. CRISPIN

1
The Human Life-Span

Good health is a condition in which both mind and body are active, alert and well nourished. Bodily and mental health are closely interwoven throughout the changing periods of our lives. The human life-span may be divided roughly as follows:

Babyhood	0–5 years
Childhood	5–13 years
Adolescence	13–20 years
Adulthood	20–45 years
Middle Age	45–65 years
Old Age	65– years

Each period is physically different from the others and the ages vary with individuals, particularly after childhood.

Babyhood

A baby is totally dependent on his mother who fulfils his basic needs of food, warmth, care and love. He sleeps nearly all the time, waking for food, for bathing and for his nappies to be changed. Mother love is very important and a baby in hospital without his mother must be cuddled and made a fuss of by a nurse.

At sixteen weeks a baby can focus his eyes on his mother, at twenty-eight weeks he can sit up without help and at about a year he can pull himself to a standing position and can crawl about.

At this age a baby is completely reliant on his mother for his cleanliness because there is no co-ordination between his voluntary brain functions and his bladder and bowels. Evacuation is merely automatic and he cannot therefore be trained to ask to use a pot until he is at least two years old and usually two and half, by which time he should be dry at night. Training is important but the baby must never be made to feel guilty if he does not learn quickly otherwise psychological difficulties may arise later.

Childhood

The arrival of a baby almost always arouses feelings of jealousy in the young child, though this may not be obvious to his mother; friends are inclined to make a great fuss of the new arrival, quite naturally, and the older child feels neglected.

By the time he is five years old and starting school he will be developing friendships with other children, learning to play with them and sharing toys, though not always willingly. He will be eating the same food as his parents, using a great deal of energy, and growing fast. He therefore needs about twelve hours sleep a day, some being taken during the day and usually after lunch.

Father also plays a very important part although as he is away working during the day he and the children do not see very much of each other. He must not become the sole awarder of punishment and reward; father and mother should always present a united front to their children.

School should be and usually is a happy place but the child is likely to return home tired and may become irritable at night; quiet games are better for him then than riotous romps. If he is worried he may revert to baby habits and even wet his bed at night.

Adolescence

The onset of puberty is usually about the age of eleven and it is at this stage that childhood ends and adolescence begins. A boy becomes more muscular and begins to grow hair on his face and body. His voice 'breaks' and becomes deeper and for a time he may not be fully in control of it. This and frequently the appearance of spots cause him embarrassment.

A girl changes too. Her approaching womanhood shows in the development of her breasts, the shapely curves of her body and the onset of menstruation.

This time is often the most difficult both for the young person and for the parents and friends. Being neither child nor adult, with changing physique and rapidly developing intelligence, to say nothing of outside pressures, the teenager is criticized and cultivated and may never be too sure of his reception. Inclined to be intolerant himself he resents controls imposed by parents, school and the law of the land. It is now that he may well decide or have decided for him the course of his entire life. Small wonder that he feels anxious and unsure, though he may hide this by being rebellious or aggressive to a greater or lesser extent.

This period of life can and often is the one in which most fun can be had, in games, trips abroad and in the learning of new skills, for it is now that lifelong interests may be started: music, dancing, painting, sailing, athletics and so on. At this age co-ordination of mind and muscle is reaching a peak.

Adulthood

The adult should be ready to accept responsibility and take initiative in his private life and chosen career and should be able to form stable relationships with others. It is natural to fall in love, to marry and to raise a family.

As members of the community, men and women can be expected to take part in local affairs by way of their church, local club, political organization or ratepayers' society. Men and women have different parts to play and both learn to adapt to circumstances, hardship or sorrow, while supporting younger or older relatives and friends.

Middle Age

People age at varying rates and in some, middle age brings to fruition the ambitions of youth. Success at work or in the family and seeing one's children growing up to independence, balance the inevitable sadness of the deaths of parents and older relatives. Physical activity declines and ideas are inclined to become fixed, though the experiences of life confer wisdom.

Physical change accompanied by endocrine change, for women the menopause, and the realization that some goals will never be reached, can make this a time of frustration and disillusionment; some find it difficult to make the necessary adjustments but now is the time to plan for retirement and old age.

Old Age

Old age is very much a state of mind but inevitably there is a slowing of mental and physical activity. Younger friends and relatives must not, with ill-judged kindness, take away too many of the responsibilities and tasks of the older person.

People live longer now in the western world though in less favoured countries old age may come in the forties or fifties. The expectation of life for men of forty has not in fact increased since 1948 which means that since women are living longer old peoples' homes are usually filled with old women. Men in general are not as strong constitutionally as women because biologically they are the more specialized member of the species and not as adaptable as women.

The retirement bungalow near the sea which is the lifelong ambition of many is sadly too often a false goal. Surrounded only by old people and seeing no children or even middle-aged friends the elderly can easily sink into bored inactivity. They make heavy demands on health and welfare services and live in an unhappy atmosphere of impending death. The south coast towns of England have become what is unkindly called the 'Costa Geriatrica'. There is a great difference between restful peace and slothful monotony. The ideal to aim for is a peaceful and dignified preparation for the end of life and this is most easily achieved in familiar surroundings.

2

Personal Health

Everyone needs and is entitled to a life in which work, rest and play are sensibly balanced. Add to these, good food and clean surroundings and you have all the ingredients of a truly healthy existence, healthy that is to say in body and in mind.

People who work for a long time in one place tend to lose their vitality and initiative; they become stagnant mentally and may easily become depressed and develop poor health.

Hospital work is always demanding especially with long term and incurable illness. A nurse must develop interests completely unconnected with her profession if she is to be of value to her patients. Many people have demanding jobs, so what is so special about nursing? The point is that men and women responsible for the safety and indeed the lives of others must live their own lives with a full awareness of that responsibility. This is also true of surgeons, airline pilots, school teachers and indeed of anyone whose mistakes or inattention can result in injury.

Rest and Sleep

After violent or prolonged exercise the muscles lose the ability to respond to the brain's instructions. You see this in the slowing down of an athlete towards the end of a long race and in your own staggering steps after climbing a long hill or staircase. Muscles use oxygen and need time to enable the blood to carry it to them to remove the lactic acid which accumulates during exercise and which can cause cramp. After a rest, when the muscles are well oxygenated, exercise can continue.

Sleep is primarily to rest the brain though as the body too is at rest the muscles also benefit. If you are very worried about an examination or the progress of one of your patients you will not sleep well because your brain will be unable to slow down its activity; for this reason you should try to sort out your worries before bedtime. If you cannot sleep you must find the reason why not both for your own and your patients' sakes. Some like to go to bed in a leisurely way, to have a bath and read a book in bed, a hot drink may soothe but you should never eat a heavy meal late in the day. Sleep is not a luxury but an absolute necessity and you should allow yourself seven or eight hours each night.

Posture

Good posture is an essential part of health, vitality and fitness. Stooping leads to poor ventilation of the lungs, round shoulders and a tendency to develop backache. Work in the ward is usually tiring though with good posture a nurse will find that she will not only be more likely to avoid back strain but also be able to perform fairly strenuous tasks in the ward more easily, e.g. lifting patients.

It is unhealthy to stand with slack muscles so that the curvature of the spine is increased and the stomach and buttocks stick out. Rather, good posture means to hold the abdomen and buttocks in (to lift the pelvic girdle), back straight, weight slightly forward on to the sides and balls of the feet and the shoulders slightly forward (to give the lungs room to fill easily). Arms and legs should be slightly flexed, not rigid and the head held up. This is how a ballet dancer stands and it should both look good and feel comfortable.

Exercise

To feel and be entirely healthy and well, it is also essential to take exercise. Babies wriggle, children play and teenagers take part in sports, but many adults take no exercise at all and many feel that because they have to stand or walk around during their work, that this is sufficient; it is not. Exercise at least two or three times a week is important, a good form of exercise being an energetic walk. With regular exercise, muscle tone is developed, the capacity of the chest and lungs is maintained and improved, appetite (as distinct from gluttony) is improved, circulation is improved and the person feels fit and contented. Constipation is prevented because peristalsis is increased, the lymphatic circulation is quickened and in every way the person is filled with a sense of well-being and his mind becomes clearer.

Personal Hygiene

Much of a nurse's work is concerned with the hygiene of her patients who, because they are ill or merely because they are in bed, cannot look after themselves. It is very important that you devote equal care to yourself as a matter of course. A daily bath and the use of a deodorant ensure that you remain fresh when you are carrying out nursing procedures in close proximity to your patient. Skin care is dealt with in detail in Chapter 28 but there are some additional points well worth mentioning.

Feet

You will be on your feet for much of the day and you may at first find this very tiring. Your feet should be washed every day and dusted lightly with talcum powder and if they have become hot with a foot powder which contains an antifungal compound. When your feet are tired and ache it is often helpful to rest with them raised above hip level and even to sleep with them on a pillow. Stockings should be washed every day. Changing them in the middle of the day and putting on another pair of shoes can be very refreshing. *Tinea pedis* (athletes' foot) can be prevented and cured by the application of foot ointment or powder and can be avoided by not using communal bathmats and by never walking barefoot even across your own bedroom.

Corns should be treated by a chiropodist though the cause of them should be removed by careful selection of properly fitting shoes; sad to say so called 'fashionable' shoes are the cause of many foot ailments and backache. Good shoes are not always dull and old-fashioned and cheap shoes are seldom a wise buy.

Flat feet can be treated by selected exercise.

Chilblains are caused by poor circulation, lack of calcium, tight shoes and by cold and damp. They are best avoided by taking exercise or massaging the feet and by wearing warm boots out of doors in cold weather. The hands too may suffer and gloves should be worn to protect them from cold wind and rain.

Ingrowing toenails are avoided by cutting the nails straight across the top with scissors; clippers are usually curved and should therefore not be used.

The hair

Your hair, whatever its style, must be brushed and combed night and morning and washed regularly and certainly once a week. After contact with a verminous patient particular attention is needed.

The bowels

Healthy living and well-balanced regular meals including fruit, green vegetables and water lead to normal bowel action. Good muscle tone from regular exercise makes it quite unnecessary to use aperients and no harm comes from not opening your bowels everyday nor at the same time each day. Aperients disturb the normal production of mucus and reduce muscle reflexes.

The monthly period

Menstruation is a natural part of a woman's life and prepares her for normal motherhood. During this time each month she should continue her normal activities suitably protected. Protection may be in the form of a pad worn externally or as a tampon worn internally. Cotton wool pads must be disposed of by being burnt and cellulose pads and tampons flushed away in the lavatory. Great care must be taken when inserting a tampon to ensure that the used one has been removed, otherwise irritation and infection may set in and a vaginal discharge ensue.

Occupational Health Services

For some time the health of nurses in hospitals has been supervised with regular medical examinations, inoculations, chest X-rays and other examinations and treatments as required. In addition most hospitals have provided medical and nursing care in illness in a special staff sick-bay. Today it is Department of Health and Social Services' policy to extend this and to have an occupational health service for all staff, not only nurses, similar to that provided in industry. This is a confidential service given by nurses specially trained for the job, and aims at keeping all staff fit and happy in their work and at minimizing any hazards to which they may be exposed while doing their jobs. It does not deal with illness which is still the province of the general medical practitioners (for non-medical staff) and the hospital nursing and medical staff. For those who are resident the occupational health nurse not only organizes and deals with medical examinations and immunization but also can often help with personal problems and anxieties on a strictly confidential basis.

Care of the Home

It is important for a house to be clean so that it is nice to look at, inside and out and healthy to live in. Bacteria thrive in dust, dirt, damp and darkness and if she can eliminate these the housewife will have done much to safeguard her family's health. Clean fresh air and sunlight are her allies and she must use them in preference to disinfectants which even in liberal amounts do little more than leave a pleasant smell.

Kitchen and larder must receive particular attention to prevent contamination of fresh food, milk and opened tins and jars. All cracked or chipped cups, plates and mixing bowls must be thrown away because they can harbour dirt and bacteria.

Bath and washbasins, need thorough cleaning with powders especially designed for them and not with very harsh scouring materials and abrasive powders which may scratch the polished surfaces and provide places for dirt to collect.

Floors must be cleaned according to their material; wooden floorboards or parquet must be polished or covered with plastic tiles or linoleum in such a way that water cannot get underneath. Particular attention is needed in the kitchen, bathroom and lavatory and wherever household pets are kept. Almost all flooring materials require polishing even the most modern ones; water and soap are normally used only to remove the most obstinate patches of dirt and if used for long periods without polish will destroy the surface of any material.

The house should be well-ventilated by regularly opening windows; scented aerosol sprays are no substitute for fresh air. Do not mask smells but get rid of their cause.

3

Aspects of Public Health

The previous chapter dealt with the health of the individual at home and at work. What we must now consider is the effect we have on our surroundings and what effect our surroundings may have on us.

When there is plenty of space for people they can choose to live where they can easily grow food and obtain water, the simplest form of existence in which the basic needs of life are met. It is interesting to see how people live nowadays when there is ample room for all. Australia, a relatively new western society, is a vast area, much of which is harsh and arid. The State of South Australia, with an area of about a million square kilometres (one tenth that of the United States or four times that of the United Kingdom), has a population of 1 200 000 which means that each person has almost a square kilometre to himself. However, this simple piece of arithmetic ignores the fact that not only do most South Australians live in towns but that three-quarters of them live in only one city, Adelaide!

In addition, despite the fact that the state produces and exports meat, wool, fruit and wine only 6 per cent of the working population works on the land. Yet in underdeveloped countries where almost everyone is a farmer, starvation is normal!

The effect of this crowding together is to prevent our looking after ourselves alone and the city, town or village has to organize itself to provide the necessary facilities of life.

Water

A constant supply of pure, drinkable water is essential for domestic and agricultural use; a factory or electricity power station will take extra measures to remove dissolved chalk from what is called 'hard' water. Water is taken from rivers, from wells and in areas of heavy rainfall from upland supplies enclosed by dams. It is stored to ensure a constant supply and also helps purification by allowing suspended impurities to sediment and by giving sunshine and wind time to perform a degree of sterilization. The water is filtered to remove any remaining matter and then sterilized with chlorine to destroy micro-organisms. The water is now safe to drink. *Fluoridation* is a means of reducing the incidence of dental caries, the rotting away of teeth. Some areas have a natural supply of fluoride in the water and it has been known for some time that people living in these areas have less dental disease.

Sewage

Human excreta form a potential source of disease and are disposed of in the sewerage system. The purpose of the system is to treat the sewage so that the end-product is clean and safe in liquid and solid form. The liquid may be disposed of in a river or, after purification, returned to the drinking water supply reservoirs. The solid is either dumped at sea or dried and used as agricultural fertilizer.

Seaside towns normally discharge their sewage directly into the sea, when the tide is receding, though in areas of dense population this easy and cheap method is causing concern. Seawater is fortunately an effective medium for dispersing and cleaning sewage.

Refuse Collection

The dry rubbish of a household is put into a dustbin outside the house and collected weekly in specially designed vehicles. Metal is removed by electromagnets and the remaining refuse burnt in great incinerators whose heat can be used to heat water for area heating schemes. Small towns usually tip their rubbish in a controlled way, care being taken to seal the tip with a layer of clean earth 22 cm (9 in) thick to keep out flies and discourage vermin such as rats.

Hospital refuse contains pathogenic micro-organisms and must therefore be burned. Soiled dressings are placed in a disposal bag and broken glass and disposable needles and syringes in another container commonly called 'the sharps box'.

Housing

Good housing makes for good health and happiness; bad housing causes bad health and misery. A home should be dry, warm and well-illuminated by both natural and artificial light. It should have a water supply and adequate and separate facilities for cooking, working and sleeping and it must have an indoor water closet. It should afford the family a degree of privacy.

Shops must be within easy reach and as far as is possible homes should be sited so as to avoid the effects of air-borne pollution, noise from factories and, much more difficult, noise from aircraft. Air-borne pollution means not only dust and smoke but smell from oil refineries and other chemical plant or food factories.

Clean Air

The air most of us breathe is quite efficiently filtered in the nose, but if the air contains very fine particles, and a great many of them, some will be drawn down to the lungs and in time cause damage which cannot be repaired and in some cases cancer of the lungs. The real dangers of breathing impure air are now well understood and in most countries there are regulations concerning the maintenance of clean air over cities. Government and Local Authority inspectors ensure that the laws are obeyed.

Factories are, whenever possible, sited down-wind from areas of housing, though this is not always a simple matter where the prevailing winds for part of the year are in one direction and at another time in the reverse direction. Nevertheless, towns are now planned with health very much in mind. It is not sufficient merely to keep homes and factories far apart because then comes the problem of people getting to work, often nowadays by car, and causing pollution as bad as that arising from the factories. Fog and its urban form, smog, are now fairly uncommon, an improvement entirely due to legislation which forbade the use of smoke-producing fuel in domestic grates and factory furnaces. To people weakened by chronic respiratory disease smog may be a killer.

4

Nutrition

Food is any substance, animal, vegetable or mineral, taken into the body to give it energy and warmth or to provide material for growth and repair. The digestive system provides the means of changing food into compounds which can be absorbed into the blood stream for transport round the body.

The normal point of entry is the mouth, though if the food must be assimilated rapidly it can be put directly into the blood stream as an intravenous infusion of dextrose, a form of sugar. If a person's upper alimentary tract has undergone extensive surgery (excision of the oesophagus for example) food may be poured directly into the stomach through an opening through the abdomen, a gastrostomy.

Essential Foods

All over the world people eat their own national dishes which are very varied in flavour and appearance. Surprisingly perhaps, they have a common basis, consisting of three main food types: carbohydrate, protein and fat. In Western Europe, for example, the basic foods are bread, meat and butter; in Italy, pasta or rice, meat and olive oil; and in India, rice or chapati, beans or meat, and butter.

Protein

This is needed for growth and repair and occurs in eggs, lean meat, pulses (beans, peas and lentils) and cereals (wheat and rye).

Carbohydrates

These provide energy and heat in the form of sugars and starches. They are found as sugars in sugar cane, sweet root vegetables (beetroot, sugar beet), honey, milk and fruits, and as starches in cereals (wheat, rice) root vegetables (potato) and pulses (beans, lentils, peas).

Fats

Fats are chemically similar to carbohydrates and serve the same purpose though they are less easy to digest and require the presence of sugar. Sources of animal fats are fish oils, cheese, yoghurt and butter. Vegetable fats are found in plant oils (olive, ground nut, coconut, sunflower and maize or sweetcorn).

Vitamins

Vitamins are organic substances which occur in many foods in very small amounts but which are essential to normal metabolism. Absence or shortage of a vitamin in the diet will produce recognizable symptoms and signs of ill-health; its addition to the diet will very quickly restore the sufferer to normal health. Vitamins are known by letters and have distinct properties.

Vitamin A strengthens resistance to infection, aids night vision and maintains healthy skin and mucous membranes. Deficiency may give rise to roughened and dry skin, inability to see in dim light and xerophthalmia leading to blindness. It is found in halibut and cod liver oil, liver, butter, cheese, eggs, carrots, spinach and tomatoes.

Vitamin B1 (thiamine) promotes the release of energy from carbohydrates. Deficiency checks growth in children, causes neuritis and also beri-beri, a severe form of neuritis, paralysis and oedema of the extremities. It is found in brewers' yeast, bacon, liver, wholemeal bread and vegetables.

Vitamin B2 (riboflavine) promotes the release of energy from carbohydrates. Deficiency checks growth, causes soreness of the lips and tongue, gives rise to digestive upsets and produces mental symptoms and pellagra. It is found in yeast, dairy produce, eggs and liver.

Vitamin B3 (nicotinic acid or niacin). The function and results of deficiency of this vitamin are the same as for vitamin B2. Sources are yeast, meat extracts, offal and wholemeal bread.

Vitamin B6 (pyridoxine) is concerned with protein metabolism. Deficiency is unlikely to occur as it is present in most foods.

Folic acid is involved in the formation of red blood cells. Deficiency results in macrocytic anaemia. Folic acid is found in liver and green vegetables.

Vitamin B12 (cyanocobalamin) is necessary for the development of red blood cells. Deficiency causes pernicious anaemia. It is found in liver, yeast, meat extracts and wholemeal bread.

Vitamin C promotes rapid healing of wounds and assists the body's resistance to infection. Necessary in growth for the formation of bones, teeth and connective tissue, it is not stored in the body and must be supplied daily. Deficiency checks growth in children, delays wound healing, causes soreness of the mouth and gums and bleeding of the capillaries and gives rise to scurvy. Sources are oranges, lemons, blackcurrants, green leaf vegetables, rosehip syrup and new potatoes.

Vitamin D enables the body to absorb calcium and phosphorus for bone and teeth. Deficiency results in rickets and osteomalacia. It can be formed by the action of ultraviolet light from the sun on the skin and it is found in halibut- and cod liver oil, egg yolk, butter, margarine, cheese and milk.

Vitamin E may have some action on the reproductive system. It is found in wheatgerm and vegetable oils, green leaves and milk.

Vitamin K is essential for the proper clotting of blood. It is found in wheatgerm, lettuce, green leaves and milk.

Mineral salts

Mineral salts are found in vegetables and meat, or in the case of table salt, eaten as the raw mineral sodium chloride, which is either dug out of salt mines or extracted from the seawater by evaporation as in tropical countries. Mineral salts are important because they contain elements which are essential for the healthy functioning of the body.

Calcium is particularly important in the formation of bone and teeth, for nerve function and also for the clotting of the blood. It is found mainly in milk and cheese and also in meat, fish and vegetables.

Sodium is present in all tissues as sodium chloride and also as sodium phosphate and sodium carbonate. It is the carbonate that makes the blood alkaline.

Iron is an essential constituent of haemoglobin because of its ready ability to combine with oxygen. Women need more than men do because of their monthly blood loss. Iron occurs in green vegetables, egg yolk and red meat.

Phosphorus is used for the building of tissues, bone and nerves. Egg yolk, milk, fish and meat are its normal sources.

Iodine is essential for the healthy functioning of the thyroid gland and is ingested from drinking water and from fish. In some areas the drinking water is deficient in iodine and the entire population may suffer from enlargement of the thyroid gland, a condition called goitre.

Milk

A human mother's milk is right for a human baby and a cow's milk is right for a calf because each milk contains nutriments in proportions best suited to the offspring it will nourish.

There are clear advantages in a mother breast-feeding her infant and this is particularly true in areas where disease flourishes. Her milk is clean and free of infective organisms, it is at the right temperature, it is readily available and in addition breast-feeding helps forge a strong emotional bond between a mother and her baby.

Milk contains protein, carbohydrate, fats, minerals, vitamins and water and therefore provides all the food that a baby needs. Unfortunately it is also an excellent breeding ground for micro-organisms and can easily be contaminated if not kept cool and covered. If a cow has tuberculosis or brucellosis the infective organisms can be transmitted in its milk and in many countries great effort has been devoted to eradicating these diseases from dairy herds. Also strict standards of cleanliness must be observed in milking parlours and people working in them must be free from illness and scrupulously clean. The cows' udders are washed before milking starts and machinery also is kept clean and sterile.

The milk is usually cooled immediately and that which is to be sold is treated and classified as follows:

Tuberculin-tested milk (T.T. Milk) is from cows certified as being free from tuberculosis. Some milk is also tested for brucellosis and if the test is negative, the milk is said to come from brucellosis-attested herds.

Pasteurized milk is milk which has been prepared in one of two ways:
1. High Temperature Short Time (HTST) when the milk is heated to 73°C (163°F) for fifteen seconds and then quickly cooled.
2. The milk is kept at between 63 and 66°C (145 and 151°F) for thirty minutes and then rapidly cooled and bottled.

Sterilized milk has been heated to 100°C (212°F) for fifteen minutes to kill bacteria.

Dried milk is milk which has been reduced to one-eighth of its bulk, all the water having been driven off by evaporation.

Dried skimmed milk is milk which has had all the cream skimmed off and removed before drying.

Evaporated milk is milk which has been reduced to one-third of its bulk by evaporation.

Condensed milk is the same as evaporated milk, but has added sugar.

Food Poisoning

Food poisoning is the result of eating contaminated cooked or uncooked fresh or preserved food. Meat products, usually made-up dishes such as meat pies, brawn and pressed beef, are the commonest cause of outbreaks. They should be kept in a cold storage unit until they are sold and then eaten soon, preferably on the same day and certainly no later than the date marked on them.

It is usual in mass catering in restaurants, schools and hospitals to cook meat, allow it to go cold and then carve it into slices for subsequent reheating, but meat pies, pork pies and all cooked meats are ordered on a daily basis.

Washing and preparation must be thorough and all cooked food should be cooked to the centre to kill micro-organisms. It is useless to cook food thoroughly after bacteria have had a chance to multiply because though cooking will sterilize the food it will not remove the toxic products which have already formed. People handling food must always wash their hands first and everyone after using the lavatory must do so.

Cracked crockery must be thrown away and customers should have the courage to refuse to eat from cracked plates in restaurants: easier said than done—but a red face is better than acute gastritis.

Calories and Obesity

The Calorie, known also as the large Calorie, kilocalorie or medical calorie, has for many years been the unit used in dietetics to measure the energy or heat-producing capacity of food. One Calorie is defined as being the amount of heat required to raise 1 kg of water 1°C; it is being replaced in dietetics by the kilojoule: 1 Calorie = 4·2 kilojoules.

Different foods have different Calorie or kilojoule values per gram, thus:

Carbohydrate	4 Cal	16·8 kJ
Protein	4 Cal	16·8 kJ
Fat	9 Cal	38 kJ
Alcohol	7 Cal	29 kJ

No Calories are provided by minerals, salts, vitamins or water.

A man in an office job needs about 2700 Cal (11 300 kJ) a day and a woman about 2200 (9000 kJ) though these amounts vary naturally with the physique of each person, with the temperature of the office and with the rate at which a person's body operates. If more food is eaten than is needed it is stored in the body; carbohydrates as glycogen in the liver, protein (part of it) as glycogen in the liver, and fat as fatty tissue all over the body. The part of protein not stored is excreted in the urine as urea. This is a simple and not completely true picture because there is a limit to the amount of sugar that can be stored but not to the amount of fat and therefore excessive amounts of sugar are converted to fat. This is another way of saying that overeating of anything is unhealthy. There is a belief that instinct will make us choose the foods most suitable to our individual needs but the great variety of foodstuffs makes it necessary for us to select what we eat very carefully. In prosperous countries we have forgotten how fundamental to life is the food we eat; it is the poor and starving who put a real value on food.

Special Diets

A 1000 calorie diet is for people who must lose weight for the sake of their health generally but especially for those with heart failure or hypertension. The patient is allowed as much undressed salad and green vegetables as he wants but his intake of protein, carbohydrate and fat is limited to 1000 Calories a day.

A high-calorie diet is given to people recovering from illness or whose weight is lower than is considered healthy. A full diet is given with extra milk and glucose but the patient is not encouraged to gorge himself at meal times.

A high-protein diet is given in malnutrition and when extensive repair of body tissue is needed, after severe burning for example.

If a patient is not eating well special foods such as Casilan or Complan may be given.

A *low-protein diet* is for people with certain kidney or liver disorders. Protein intake is restricted to a specified amount but to prevent breakdown of body protein consumption of carbohydrates and fats is encouraged. Peas, beans and lentils are not allowed but other vegetables and fruit may be eaten.

A *low-fat diet* is prescribed for patients with jaundice or inflammation of the gall bladder (cholecystitis). This entails the avoidance of butter, fat meat, herrings, sardines, pastries and puddings, nuts, egg yolk and salad cream and no fried food is allowed.

A *low-salt diet* is for patients with congestive heart failure and severe hypertension accompanied by oedema. No salt is used in cooking and all salty foods and those containing baking powder are restricted. The aim is to reduce sodium intake.

A *gluten-free diet* is essential for patients with coeliac disease. Gluten is the protein in some cereals, namely wheat, barley and rye, and these and their products must never be eaten. Cereals or cereal-type products which do not contain gluten are rice, sago, soya flour, tapioca, potato flour and cornflakes. Many foods contain cereals even though this may not be obvious, and among these are sausages, sauces, soups, sweets and the following drinks: Bengers, Horlicks and Ovaltine.

A *diabetic diet* is for those people who cannot metabolize sugar and starch without the administration of insulin either orally or by subcutaneous injection.

5

Household Pests and Parasites

A parasite is an animal or vegetable organism which depends for its existence on another living thing. Pests are those creatures of the animal kingdom that we do not want in our homes. They may wish to live with us but they do not live on us. Parasites may be insects (six-legged and with head, body and tail segments), arachnids (eight-legged ticks, mites), worms or moulds.

Some pests and parasites occur all over the world while others are restricted to particular areas.

The Housefly

The fly cannot eat solid food but first dissolves it with saliva which it spits on to the food and then sucks up. Vomiting and defaecating while it eats, the fly contaminates more food with micro-organisms whilst the hairs on its body continually collect and shed dust. The following points are important in *prevention*:

(1) Cover dustbins with well-fitting lids and ensure regular cleaning and disinfection.

(2) See that rubbish is removed frequently. It takes only eight days for a fly to develop from its egg.

(3) Keep all food covered and when laying tables, place crockery upside down until it is used.

(4) Cover larder windows with fine wire-netting so that fresh air can circulate but flies cannot enter.

(5) Compost and manure heaps must be kept well away from the house.

The Mosquito

The cause of worldwide misery, the mosquito sucks blood and may transmit disease (malaria, yellow fever, elephantiasis). In countries where it is a disease carrier the people should protect their bodies by wearing clothes which completely cover them (shirts buttoned at the wrist and long trousers) and by sleeping in beds guarded by sleeping nets. Windows are covered by fine screens.

Insect Parasites

The head louse

The head louse is a little light-greyish insect which lays its eggs, known as nits, in hard cases and glues them into its host's head near the roots of the hair. The eggs hatch in about ten days and the lice immediately begin to cause irritation by sucking blood.

Head lice are destroyed by the application of one of the proprietary preparations containing an insecticide. They are applied to the hair and scalp, left for a few hours and then washed out. Old-fashioned remedies, carbolic acid and sassafras oil, are used only when modern products are unobtainable.

The body louse

This louse is similar in appearance to the head louse though its colour changes according to the colour of hair of its victim. Usually found on unclean and elderly people, the nits are attached to clothing. Clothing must be fumigated and the patient given a hot bath and afterwards the appropriate ointment is applied to the affected parts of the body and where necessary the body hair is shaved.

Many diseases are caused by lice, among them typhus fever which is fortunately almost unknown in Britain. Nurses who protect themselves from lice by wearing protective clothing and have good health seldom contract typhus.

The flea

The flea has a horny brown hard outer covering and very large, strong back legs which enable it to jump several feet. The eggs are laid in cracks and crevices of a dirty room and take about nineteen days to develop. Infected rooms and furniture must be fumigated by the Local Authority and all dust burned. In some hot countries there is a variety of flea which sucks the blood of plague-infected rats and then transmits it to humans.

The bed bug

This is a flat, oval, brownish insect which lays its eggs in clusters in the cracks in old walls, floors and furniture. The eggs mature in about a week. Fumigation can be achieved only by the use of a poisonous gas in empty premises and only by trained operators.

Arachnids

Ticks, mites, spiders, and scorpions

These are not insects because they have eight legs. In Britain ticks and mites commonly live on cattle and domestic pets and may be transferred to humans. Scorpions live only in hot climates, vary in colour from pale brown to black and carry a dangerous poisonous sting in the tail.

The itch-mite (Sarcoptes scabiei). This is a round, white, shiny, eyeless mite, just visible to the naked eye. It burrows into thin parts of the skin such as the crevices of fingers, toes and elbows, lays its eggs and then seals them up by means of a sticky fluid which it deposits all over the skin.

Treatment consists of gently scrubbing open the burrows after a hot bath and killing the mite by applying a preparation of benzyl benzoate emulsion. This is allowed to dry for about twenty minutes before the patient gets dressed in freshly laundered clothes. All clothing and bed linen must be fumigated before it is washed and mattresses must also be fumigated. The patient's bedstead must be washed with hot soapy water and disinfected. Some people become hypersensitive to the itch-mite and develop a generalized skin rash four to six weeks later.

Rats

Rats may carry plague, food poisoning, worms and jaundice as well as being a danger to children and pets whom they may attack. The Local Authority should be told when a rat has been seen and a trained operator will then deal with this menace to health.

Worms

Threadworms

Threadworms appear in the stools as little white threads, pointed at each end. They may be contracted by drinking infected water or by eating carelessly prepared vegetables. In Western Europe tap water is normally clean and free from infective organisms, but where there is any reason to doubt the quality of water it must be boiled before being drunk. Children are most commonly infested and may reinfest themselves because the worm eggs are laid on the skin around the anus. They soon dry and are freely scattered in clothes, on floors and on furniture; the child scratches and carries the eggs to his mouth on his fingers. While being treated this must be prevented by applying a soothing ointment to the anus, lightly splinting the arms at night and putting the child to sleep in pyjamas.

Roundworms

Similar to the earthworm though paler, they are 15–41 cm (6–16 in) long. Like the threadworm they may be found in infected water and vegetables. They wander about the body causing disease and obstruction and may be vomited from the stomach or passed in the stools. Symptoms are abdominal pain and in some cases, convulsions.

Tapeworms

These may be many feet long and consist of a head and a body made up of segments in which eggs develop. These segments break off from the head without killing the worm. The usual source of infestation is meat, usually pork or beef, and also fish which has not been throughly cooked through. The head of the worm is usually embedded high up in the small intestine, the body taking up space in the intestinal tract and absorbing a great deal of the person's food. Treatment is by drugs, prescribed by the doctor and taken by mouth. Stools may have to be examined until the doctor is satisfied that the head of the worm has been passed and the patient is cured.

Ringworm

Ringworm or tinea is not a worm but the name given to a vegetable mould which attacks the scalp or the skin of the body. The mould forms spores which may blow about and spread the infection wherever they settle. Pets may be a means of spreading the complaint and a veterinary surgeon should be consulted.

Treatment is by antibiotic drug given by mouth and by applying fungicidal ointments to the affected areas. Clothes must be changed daily and hats must have a washable lining. Everything used by the patient must be disinfected.

6

Accidents at Home

With care and forethought most accidents in the home could be avoided. Yet every year in Britain more people are killed at home than in traffic accidents. Those most at risk are the very young and the elderly.

General Safety

Old people's failing eyesight, lack of agility and poor sense of balance make them particularly liable to accidents caused by falling over obstacles and stumbling on steps and stairs. All rooms, passages and landings must be well lit in such a way that there are no deep shadows to conceal small tables or chairs. Stairs need firm handrails, and stair carpets must be securely fixed with no loose ends to trip on. Floors must never be slippery and small mats, particularly in doorways, must never be used. Light switches must be easily situated and stair-way lights switched on or off from both the foot and the top of the stairs.

For children's safety there should be a gate at the top of the stairs or across the nursery door and all open fires must be guarded with a spark-proof screen.

Electrical Hazards

All electrical equipment must be treated with great care because an electric shock can burn or kill. Badly maintained plugs and switches and frayed flex are a fire hazard as well.

Some electrical machinery is fully insulated and has a two-wire flex while other machinery is earthed and has a three-wire flex and three-pin plugs. A professional electrician should be responsible for installation and can tell you which system is appropriate. Electric fires and irons always have an earth wire, though television sets and electric drills are often fully insulated. There is an added advantage in the three-wire earthed system using shutter plugs: a safety shutter covers the live terminals which only lift when a plug with an earth terminal is inserted and this prevents children pushing screwdrivers into the live sockets.

In the bathroom even greater care is necessary because water is a good conductor of electricity and steam may condense into switches and electrical elements. A radiant electric heater may be installed if the element is sealed in silica (a form of glass) and if the whole unit is firmly fixed in place above head level so that it cannot be touched accidentally either by hand or by a damp towel. The immersion heater must not have a switch in the bathroom and no switch may be within reach of the bath. For added safety pull cord switches should be used.

Electrical hazards in the kitchen are the same as those in the bathroom. Again water, being a good conductor of electricity, is a particular hazard with the added danger from cooking stove hot-plates which can become very hot but not so hot as to glow red and be seen.

During thunderstorms outdoor television and radio aerials should be unplugged because they can conduct lightning which will not only destroy the set but may scatter the contents of the set around the room with explosive force.

Household Gas

Cookers, convection heaters, open gas fires and water heating boilers are potentially dangerous as fire hazards and as sources of asphyxiating gas. Coal gas, natural gas and bottled gas need the same amount of attention to certain details. All rooms with gas installations must be well-ventilated and no one should sleep in a room in which a gas heater is left burning.

Modern gas cookers have a pilot light which burns continually and lights the main burners or oven when they are turned on. Older cookers and fires are lit with a match and for safety the match must be lit before the gas is turned on, otherwise, particularly in an oven, the gas can accumulate before being lit and may possibly cause an explosion.

Safety in the Kitchen

The kitchen contains many sources of injury in addition to electrical ones: boiling water for vegetables (100°C (212°F)), a pressure cooker (122°C (252°F)) and frying oil or fat (205°C (401°F)). Compare these temperatures with that for a baby's bath (38°C (100°F)) and you can see that great care must be taken to protect children by keeping them out of the kitchen and by turning all saucepan handles so that they do not extend over the sides of the cooker.

Knives, cleavers, mincers and mixers provide temptation for children and are best kept out of sight.

Oil Heaters and Lamps

Oil heaters are still a cause of serious domestic accidents. They are basically of two types, those in which the flame is enclosed in a glass or metal funnel and those in which it is open. Unfortunately it is those with an open flame which give off the greatest amount of heat; in addition the oil is fed by gravity from an inverted container which means that if there is a breakage or leak oil will flow freely over the floor.

Heaters with enclosed flames are markedly safer because the flame cannot be touched by a flapping nightdress or dressing gown and because the oil is burnt from a wick which sucks upwards. Usually the body of the heater is made of metal which further isolates the flame so that even the hot funnel cannot be touched inadvertently; this type of heater usually extinguishes if it is knocked over and even then the oil can escape only through the wick.

No oil heater should stand in a draught nor where an opening door will cause a draught even momentarily. The flame must be extinguished when the heater is to be moved or filled.

Oil heaters are usually a cheaper source of heat than electric fires or electric radiators; they are therefore most often used by the poorer members of the community who live in the worst conditions. Burning oil gives off water vapour which increases the dampness of ill-ventilated rooms.

Oil-burning lamps are a source not only of light but of heat, and their glass funnels become so hot as to cause a severe burn and the heat above the funnel is so intense that a cigarette can be lit a full 50 cm (18 in) above it.

Medicines and Household Chemicals

All medicinal products should be kept in a locked cupboard out of reach of children, and drugs no longer required should be thrown away down the lavatory, not in the dustbin. Many drugs nowadays are produced in highly coloured capsules and closely resemble sweets. Bleaches, fly sprays and disinfectants should also be out of the reach of children and empty containers must never be given to children to play with.

The Garden and Garage

Never keep a pesticide or weedkiller in any bottle but the one it was bought in; children recognize a fruit juice bottle even when the label has been removed and may drink the contents with terrible consequences.

Stakes for plants are a common cause of serious eye injury. Rotary lawn mowers, which can throw out stones at a very high speed and whose cutting blades can and have cut off toes, must be used with care on clear grass only.

Car engines must not be left running when the car is in its garage and the car must never be backed into the garage or the poisonous carbon monoxide gas from the exhaust may accumulate. The ignition keys must not be left in the ignition socket or a child may play with them and start the engine.

7

The Nurse in the Community

Nurses fill several widely different roles in the community and additionally, they fill them in widely differing communities. A large part of the work of these nurses is only distantly connected with care of the sick, being a preventive role and the fostering of positive health. Looking around we see them working as district nurses or, as they are now often called, practice nurses, as health visitors, as public health nurses, as occupational health nurses, and as community psychiatric nurses. The exact nature of their jobs varies very considerably, some are mainly clinical, some preventive and some contain elements of both but these nurses have one thing in common, they have all received a full general training. The learning of basic skills is behind them although they may still be learning new skills for their specialist role in the community.

Let us now look in more detail at nurses working in the community where no less than ninety per cent of all illness is treated.

The Health Visitor

The Health Visitor must be state registered and either be a qualified midwife or hold an approved obstetric certificate. Her community training consists of an academic year at a university or a polytechnic followed by three months of supervised practice. There is a written examination and report on practice. Success in both qualifies her for the certificate of the Central Council for the Training of Health Visitors. Her work is non-clinical and her role a preventive and supportive one. She is responsible for all age groups 'from the womb to the tomb', although she has certain statutory responsibilities towards the newly-born and the under-fives. She is a practitioner in her own right although, obviously, she discusses and consults with colleagues not only in her own discipline but in medicine and social work. She has no legal right of entry to a home and so her acceptance by the families for whom she is responsible is one she must build and work at patiently without becoming discouraged by failure or rebuffs.

In the structure of the National Health Service she works for the District Health Authority and is managed administratively by a nursing officer. She is, herself, responsible for her own standards of practice and the management of her caseload. The essence of her work is long-term and she may see the results of this work only over a period of many years or even in a second generation.

At one time health visiting was a profession followed exclusively by women but the last few years have seen the opening up of more opportunities for men and an increasing number of them are finding this work rewarding and satisfying and many patients are benefiting from their entry into this branch of the nursing profession.

The Public Health Nurse

This group of nurses may be given a number of different titles but the essential nature of their work is much the same whatever the title. In effect they assist the health visitor with the less specialized aspects of her work. They may be state registered or enrolled and, obviously, the level of their work varies according to their level of qualification, but it has elements of both the clinical and the preventive. There is no specific national training but they are prepared by way of indoctrination courses and continuing in-service training.

In assisting the health visitor much of their work is in the school health service, assisting at periodic and special medical inspections or health surveys, dealing with minor ailments of schoolchildren or assisting with the nursing care of severely handicapped children in special schools. They also assist the health visitor with routine visiting at her discretion.

Public health nurses work for the District Health Authority. Their professional responsibility is to the health visitor and they are managed by a nursing officer.

The District Nurse

The District nurse may be registered or enrolled. Ideally she should hold the National Certificate of District Nursing but this is not, at present, mandatory. The course for this is taken at an approved training centre and consists of classroom teaching, visits for observation and field work experience. Examination is by a written paper and on-going assessment. The registered nurse takes a four-month course (reduced to three months for midwives and health visitors); the enrolled nurse takes a ten-week course.

District nursing is the only section of the community nursing services that has a mainly clinical role, although, even here, the nurse is still concerned with preventive work and health education.

At the present time district nursing, of all sections of nursing, is probably undergoing the most radical changes in concept and practice. Traditionally district nurses worked with patients in their own homes, their caseloads covered a geographical area and their clinical responsibility was to any doctor treating a patient in that area who asked for their services. In some parts of the country this pattern persists, but, increasingly, the district nurse is a specialist member of a primary care team. She gives nursing care to all patients needing care who are the responsibility of a particular medical practice and this care may be given in their own homes or at surgery clinics. She acts as nursing adviser to the primary care team and may, herself, head a nursing team of other registered and enrolled nurses and auxiliaries in the same way as does the ward sister in hospital.

It has been said of the district nurse that she 'nurses not a patient but a family, not a family but a community' and that she 'teaches without seeming to teach'. She is responsible for the total nursing care of her patients, i.e. physical, mental, emotional, spiritual, social and financial, and must take all these factors into account when planning nursing care and in advising, helping and supporting her patients.

She is clinically responsible to the general practitioner, is managed by a nursing officer and works for the District Health Authority. Her actual clinical work can encompass almost any field of nursing although she will not, in practice, usually have much contact with immediate postoperative care after major surgery. She will, however, increasingly be dealing with patients involved in early discharge schemes who have returned home early in their recovery from such surgery. In addition many primary care teams undertake minor surgery within the practice and the nurse will, of course, have her own specialized function in this.

In her actual practice she cannot, of course, develop stereotyped work methods applicable to all situations. Homes differ, facilities differ, needs differ and, moreover people differ. In every new situation she must first assess need and then plan to meet this need. The planning must be not only immediate but long-term, reaching forward to the ultimate end of the nursing situation as far as she can foresee it. At the same time her planning must be sufficiently flexible to allow for possible variations in conditions and circumstances. In order to function in this way the district nurse must develop the ability to break down basic skills so that, in the process of adapting to varied situations her techniques still fulfil professional criteria. Thus, in the comparatively simple process of bathing a patient, she may help him into a fixed bath or into a portable 'bungalow bath', wheel him in a wheelchair into a shoulder height shower cabinet or a Medibath, bath him in bed or in a chair by the fire. But, however different the situation, she still will observe the basic principles of bathing, respecting a patient's modesty, using the opportunity of gently mobilizing all limbs and observing his physical condition. She will also be noting the warmth of his surroundings, the availability and suitability of clothing, nutrition, the maintenance or deterioration of sight and hearing, of personal habits and all evidence of physical well-being or otherwise. In addition she will, tactfully and unobtrusively, be exploring any possible problems that the patient may have whether it be physical, emotional, social or financial. If such problems exist the nurse will not try to offer ready-made solutions but encourage the patient to work through to these himself. In this, of course, the district nurse can call on the resources of both statutory and voluntary social services where appropriate.

The description of the work of the district nurse has so far dealt more with the registered than the enrolled nurse although in many ways it is applicable to both. The enrolled nurse has her place as a member of the primary care team. She is totally responsible for her own standards of care but the assessment of need and the taking of decisions on levels of care and care planning are the responsibilities of the registered nurse to whom the enrolled nurse relates in the team. She will, of course, discuss plans with the enrolled nurse and bring her in on the execution of them.

However, the enrolled nurse has considerable freedom and therefore considerable responsibility, perhaps sometimes almost more than she can deal with and her point of reference, whether it be the general practitioner or registered nurse, may be distant geographically or temporarily inaccessible. This last point emphasizes a fact which nurses may find at once both frightening and challenging. This is that, except when the nurse is actually working in the practice surgery she has no access to professional support at the moment and the point of need. She may be called on to make decisions that are sometimes only marginally within her province or, if within her professional competence, may have to be made without time for considering alternatives.

The Community Psychiatric Nurse

This community worker will be discussed in Chapter 8 because of the very close liaison needed with specialist hospitals rather than practice teams and because the job of the community psychiatric nurse is so comparatively new that, in many cases, the role is still unclarified.

The Occupational Health Nurse

Any account of community nursing would not be complete without mentioning the work of the occupational health nurse. It is a matter for regret that in the 1974 restructuring of the National Health Service the opportunity was not taken of bringing within it a comprehensive occupational health service to serve the whole of the working population.

Standards of occupational health services vary from those offering little more than first aid to sophisticated services employing, as well as company medical officers and trained occupational health nurses, dentists, chiropodists, opticians and social workers. In such progressive forward-looking services the nurse will hold a Certificate of Occupational Health Nursing in addition to her state registration. Here the nurse's role is not only of merely manning a surgery; rather she spends a good deal of her time, as does the industrial medical officer, in moving about all working areas identifying health hazards such as bad lighting, poor working postures, unhealthy working conditions, absence of safety measures and preventible stress, both physical and mental. She instigates and carries out positive health programmes from, for instance, regular chest X-rays for workers in damp or dusty conditions to complete health checks at frequent intervals for all senior executives subject to stress hazards. She may visit sick workers at home either alone or with a member of the personnel and welfare department, not to spy on the worker but to see if there is any help needed to aid recovery that the firm might be able to provide.

The occupational health nurse has a very difficult course to steer between on the one hand being thought to be a tool of the management and on the other, of over-identification with the labour force. All parties must feel free to talk to her without fear of betrayal, yet she must be able to focus attention on and insist on action on working practices likely to lead to injury or illness, and therefore to loss of productivity, from whichever source that particular practice originates. She must be able to distinguish the genuine from the malingerer and any mistake she makes may cost her employer a great deal of money either as compensation or by industrial action. Her job, too, may call for reserves of physical courage and stamina. Nurses have been at the coal face in pit accidents, in smelting shops and forges, in the holds of cargo ships and working under compression conditions in tunnelling and diving operations.

Finally there are the nurses working in schools and colleges, sometimes nursing sick students, counselling, advising and maintaining positive health. We should not forget, too, the nurses who staff Family Planning Clinics and, in some areas, the Domiciliary Family Planning Service. Their work, although requiring clinical skills, involves much more than that if they are to meet the needs of their clients.

The nursing practised in the community is predominantly concerned with the prevention of illness and the maintenance of positive health. Where nurses are concerned with caring for the sick their patients tend to be approaching the end of life, either the very old or the terminally ill, or those suffering severe long-term sickness or disablement. It is no denigration of their role to say that the hospital's bed-occupancy could be considerably shortened and their waiting lists reduced if more use were made of these highly trained nursing experts and their excellent back-up services, by means of early discharge schemes of patients suffering from acute illnesses. Perhaps, in the future, we shall see more Health Care Planning Teams directed towards this end.

8

Mental Illness

In Great Britain today about half the beds in hospitals are occupied by the mentally ill and many thousands of people are treated as hospital out-patients or by their family doctors for some form of mental illness. In fact, about one in every nine women and one in every fourteen men will have some form of psychiatric illness during their lives, if the current state of affairs persists. In the light of such factors there is now an increasing awareness of mental health among the community today and demands for effective treatment of mental illness mean that this area of medicine is in great need of skilled and understanding nursing staff. This chapter is designed to give a broad understanding of the situation.

Mental illness has long been recognized, although it has not always been regarded as an illness. In ancient times mental illness was looked at with fear and superstition, the work of devils and demons and even in more recent times ill people have been treated cruelly by their neighbours. Witchcraft provided a convenient explanation. Towards the end of the nineteenth century, when the local government authorities were made responsible for the mentally sick, a large number of institutions, or asylums, were built in remote country areas to house them. The solution to a difficult problem seemed to consist of taking the awkward customers and hiding them away in the country, far from their homes and families, so that they might cause no trouble and could be safely forgotten about. Conditions in those institutions were not pleasant and a great deal of fear was associated with them. As a result it was considered a shameful thing to have relatives in them, and even more shameful to be inside oneself. This atmosphere, combined with lack of knowledge of how mental illness came about and difficulty in treating it, explains how mental hospitals simply provided custodial care for patients and very little of the therapeutic environment needed for them. The stigma associated with mental illness is only slowly breaking down even today.

In 1959 the Mental Health Services Act became law and the

mental health services of Great Britain entered a new era. All previous laws relating to mental illness were repealed and people were now able to enter psychiatric hospitals for treatment in the same way as other patients are admitted to any general hospital. This was a great break with past tradition and now over ninety-five per cent of people receiving treatment in psychiatric hospitals are 'informal' patients, which means that they are there of their own free will. The act does make provision for compulsory admission to hospital for people who may be a danger to themselves or to others and some are also referred to hospital care from the courts or prisons or brought to hospital by the police. There are obvious dangers in a system that allows people to be put into hospital against their wishes, so certain safeguards are built into the Act to ensure that people who are so detained, and their families, may have the right to appeal against this detention.

For a comprehensive understanding the nurse is advised to read the whole of the Mental Health Services Act, though Sections 25, 26, 29, 30 and 136 are those she will most frequently refer to while working in a general hospital or in the community.

Different Kinds of Mental Illness

There are many kinds of mental illness and when the nurse reads further books she will find that there are also many ways of describing and classifying them.

In this section a list of the more common types of mental illness will be given and the main features of the illness described so that some guide to understanding may be achieved. The nurse would do well to remember, however, that mental illness may present in many different ways and often features of different illnesses may be present in the same patient, producing a bewildering picture.

To understand the subject there are a few technical words which are useful to know and the following list gives these words and a description of their meaning:

Organic disorders are illnesses in which the patient has some known physical cause for the symptoms of his illness. This may be an infectious disease with high temperature, a brain tumour or destruction of some of the brain cells.

Functional disorders are illnesses in which there are no known physical causes for the patient's symptoms, for example, in depression or schizophrenia.

Delusion is a false belief which is held with conviction and cannot be changed by appeal to reason. In addition, the belief is out of character with the patient's cultural and educational background. For example, a patient may believe that he is the King of England which is obviously a delusion. However, many delusions are not so obvious and a nurse should be aware of this.

Hallucinations are sensory perceptions which have no external stimulus. The patient may hear voices when no-one else is around, or he may see things that no-one else can see. This is important for the nurse to understand because she may be the first person to observe hallucinations in a patient. She should also remember that these experiences are very real to the patient and may be frightening as well.

Neurosis means an illness in which the patient is aware that he is ill or has problems that require help and treatment. He may not understand the exact nature of his illness, but he does have some understanding or 'insight'.

Psychosis refers to an illness in which the patient is out of contact with reality and is the state that is often called 'madness'. The patient may deny that he is ill, and possibly regard efforts to treat him as part of a plot against him.

Insight is a term used to describe the patient's awareness of his own illness or problems and is associated with understanding.

Some Mental Illnesses

Acute confusional states

Acute confusional states may be associated with a number of conditions, such as fever, poisoning with drugs, kidney failure, diabetes mellitus and heart failure, in which shortage of oxygen to the brain aggravates the patient's illness. This condition is very common in hospital and is usually short-lived, being cured by successful treatment of the underlying disorder. The patient is restless, may not know where he is, especially at night and may also have delusions that he is being ill-treated or has been kidnapped. Very commonly the patient has hallucinations, especially 'seeing things'. His memory is poor and he is often overactive and unable to co-operate with the nurses. For example, he may pull out intravenous infusions or pull up naso-oesophageal tubes. Besides these features the underlying illness will present its own symptoms, such as rapid pulse and breathing or a high temperature.

Dementia

Dementia is an organic state in which there is destruction of brain cells leading to the characteristic signs of the illness. This destruction may be caused by excessive alcoholic intake or drugs such as barbiturates in excessive doses, or it may be due to no known cause. If dementia occurs before the age of sixty it is called presenile dementia and is frequently the result of drugs or alcohol.

The patient will suffer from a general intellectual 'falling off' and will have disturbance of memory associated with disorientation. He may also have changes of mood and show swings from depression to happiness. Finally there may also be changes in behaviour resulting in social embarrassment. The onset of the illness is gradual and unfortunately, because the brain cells are destroyed, cannot be cured, although some training may help to overcome a few of the problems. Gradual loss of memory occurs and failure to remember recent events is common. The patient forgets why he went out of the house and loses things he has put down and to compensate for this may make up a story to describe what he has done to account for his time. This is called confabulation. It is important to remember that this is not a question of telling lies. The story is told because the patient really believes it and he is not aware that it is inaccurate.

Neglect of personal hygiene and neglect of dressing may be a very distressing symptom for the family, and the rapid changes of mood may be very difficult for the relatives to cope with. The patient's confusion and disorientation may result in wandering about at night or getting lost in the street during the day. In hospital nurses may be mistaken by the patient for his own family and are often addressed by the names of his own children or grandchildren.

Depression

Depression is a state that many of us experience at some time or another, but a depressive illness is a much more serious and disabling illness and one that nurses will frequently encounter in hospital wards. They may see it in patients who have been admitted with a physical illness and in those who have attempted to end their lives by suicide. Depression may be precipitated by some obvious event in a patient's life, such as failing an examination, the break-up of a friendship, or the death of a close relative or friend. Alternatively there may be no obvious external event before the onset of the illness. The patient can be a man or woman of any age, although depression is more common amongst older people than amongst the young.

The signs and symptoms are:

(1) General slowing of activity, loss of appetite, constipation.

(2) Disturbance of sleep, the patient either having difficulty in getting off to sleep, or else waking very early and not going to sleep again.

(3) Expression of a sense of unworthiness, deserving to be punished.

(4) Loss of concentration which may lead to inability to manage at work.

(5) Feelings of hopelessness about the future, suicidal thoughts, or actual attempts to kill himself.

(6) Loss of contact with friends, family and work, leading to isolation.

Anxiety states

Anxiety is a feeling which is common to everyone and is often a very useful emotion in the correct measure, helping people to be aware of their surroundings and often enabling them to get things done. How often is the anxiety caused by an examination a spur to work to pass that examination? Like many good things too much anxiety is harmful and can cause much misery and suffering.

Anxiety states may be characterized by a permanent state of fear of some impending doom, either to the patient or to those close to him, which is not related directly to reality. For example, fear of being knocked over by a car in the street. This is something that does happen to many, but most people are not housebound by the fear that if they go out they will be knocked down! Not infrequently the anxiety may be fixed to a particular object or animal and in this case is called a phobia. There are endless examples of phobias and people have been reported as phobic of cats, dogs, mice, spiders, snakes and birds and of many other situations such as being in confined or open spaces.

A common result of anxiety states is that the patient uses rituals to try and control his anxiety and displays obsessional behaviour. For example, elaborate checks are made on doors, gas taps and electric switches, often in a special order and if anything is out of place the whole sequence must be repeated. A second common ritual is related to the patient's fear of being dirty or contaminated and this results in elaborate cleaning of the patient's own body, especially hands and anything with which he may come into contact.

The patient will show the physical signs of anxiety such as rapid pulse, sweating, possibly diarrhoea, loss of appetite and indigestion, and will complain of feeling tense and frightened of some unknown fear or danger or possibly of a specific phobia.

Anxiety states often accompany some depressive illness, and usually cause domestic and social upheavals in the life of the patient and his family.

Hysteria. In psychiatry the term hysteria is not used to describe crying and shouting as it is in everyday life. Hysteria is a disorder which is incapacitating for the patient because it is his means of resolving internal conflicts of which he is usually unaware. This means of resolution of conflict can be frustrating for those around the hysterical patient because they can usually see the situation more clearly than he can.

Hysteria affects males as well as females, and can manifest its symptoms in many ways, although the main principles of the patient appearing relatively unconcerned *belle indifference*, and the presence of a 'secondary gain' or advantage to the patient can usually be seen. Thus hysteria may present as loss of memory, paralysis of arms or legs, loss of speech, blindness or deafness. A simple example of hysteria is seen in the mother who has angry feelings towards a small child and wants to hit the child; she may feel guilty about this and the ensuing conflict may be resolved by 'paralysis' of the arm. Thus the problem is resolved because the mother is not now able to hit the child and, indeed, she herself requires help to treat her 'paralysed' arm.

In many cases hysteria can be confused with organic disorders such as brain tumours and the diagnosis should never be made lightly and without thorough investigation.

Anorexia nervosa. Anorexia nervosa is a state which tends to affect young people rather than older people and is much more common in females than males. The disorder frequently starts at puberty and consists of a refusal to take food which may start as an initial desire to slim which then gets out of control. The patient loses weight, may take purgatives to reduce weight further and may induce vomiting after eating, especially if pressure is brought to bear by parents to enforce eating. In girls menstruation usually ceases. In spite of obvious weight loss the patient insists she is still fat and often remains cheerful and surprisingly active.

The condition can result in death and is therefore a serious problem. The refusal to eat is associated with disturbances and conflict in relationships between parents, especially mother and the affected child and this disturbance is usually considered to be a part of the illness. These problems usually mean that the patient requires treatment in hospital in order to regain weight and the co-operation of parents is an essential part of the treatment programme involving drugs and psychotherapy.

The schizophrenias

Schizophrenia is the mental illness that is most feared and least understood by the public. This is because in this group of illnesses the patients may have periods of loss of contact with reality and demonstrate all the signs of 'madness' which can be frightening for him, his family and observers.

There are many theories about the cause of schizophrenia. Some say that it is biochemical or hereditary, others that it is not an illness at all but a form of adaptation to a difficult family life and the truth may well be a mixture of these ideas. The illness may occur at any time of life but often makes its first appearance in young people who may be affected on and off over a long period of time. Schizophrenia used to be an illness that consigned sufferers to a lifetime in a mental hospital, but today treatment with drugs means that many patients can lead a life outside hospital and very few now become chronic hospital inhabitants. They can be treated with drugs and tranquillizers and remain in the community at home and at work.

What is schizophrenia? It is not a Dr Jekyll and Mr Hyde type of condition that many people imagine. It is an illness in which the patient loses contact with reality, has difficulty in thinking properly and has great difficulty in establishing human relationships and mixing with other people. When talking to a patient with schizophrenia the nurse may get the feeling that she is not 'getting through' to him.

The patient also loses interest in his appearance and neglects personal hygiene during acute attacks of illness. Strange ideas may be expressed in the form of delusions or hallucinations; the patient may say that he is persecuted by his neighbours, that his thoughts are being influenced by waves from the television, or that part of his body is dead. He will not be confused about where he is, although he may misinterpret the hospital as a place where he is in danger of being harmed rather than helped. He may suffer from memory lapses when he is speaking and suddenly stop in mid-sentence and seem lost in space. This is called 'thought blocking'. In speech he may also make up nonsense words which may have some significance to him but are not intelligible to listeners.

Manic–depressive psychosis

This is a condition in which periods of depressive illness alternate with periods of mania. The periods of depression (p. 37) tend to last longer than the manic ones.

Manic episodes consist of overactive behaviour and the patient operates both physically and mentally at a very fast pace. This means that he tends to move about a great deal, complains of feeling hot, does not sit down to eat or drink and talks a lot, with thoughts flying from one topic to another very quickly. A patient in a manic state may give away money or valuables, make purchases beyond his means and get into serious financial troubles without realizing what he is doing.

This can be very tiring for the people around the patient. He does not tire easily and can be very difficult to occupy as his concentration is poor and his level of tolerance of frustration is low. He can become angry if thwarted in what he wants to do.

Personality or behaviour disorders

These are a wide group of conditions in which the patient does not suffer from any clearly defined mental illness but nevertheless has problems of such a kind as to cause serious disruption of his emotional, social and working relationships. The exact causes of these disorders are unknown but it is generally thought that early experiences are of some importance, especially the years of childhood development.

Many forms of sexual deviation may result from personality disorders, examples being some forms of homosexuality, transvestism (dressing in clothes appropriate to the opposite sex to obtain sexual satisfaction) and fetishism (use of articles of clothing, such as shoes, as objects for sexual gratification).

Abuse of drugs is another common aspect of personality disorder. The main drug used in Great Britain is alcohol, though there is now some concern about abuse of drugs such as heroin, cocaine, cannabis, methedrine, barbiturates and amphetamines among the young.

Psychopathy is a form of mental disorder recognized by the Mental Health Act 1959 in which the patient finds it difficult to form relationships with any warmth or depth and although the intellect is not impaired the psychopath seems to find it difficult to learn from experience. Thus antisocial behaviour tends to be repeated. The psychopath is impulsive and self-centred, finding frustration difficult to cope with and he may respond angrily or aggressively to disappointments that may seem trivial to an outside observer.

Dealing with the Problem—Treatment

Before discussing the different types of treatment available to patients suffering from mental illness mention should be made of the importance of teamwork in the approach to the patient. The therapeutic team includes nurses, doctors, occupational therapists, social workers, and psychologists as well as workers in the community such as the Disablement Resettlement Officer who helps to find suitable work. At any given time in treatment any one of the above may be the most important person for the patient, but without teamwork the patient would most certainly suffer.

Psychotherapy

This means treatment by talking with a doctor or another therapist about the patient's feelings. This can be done individually or in groups, and for many patients this is the most important part of their treatment, since it enables them to understand many of the problems which have been besetting them, and so leads to their solution.

Drug therapy

There are many drugs used to treat mental illness but they fall into three main categories:

Antidepressants. These drugs cause a change of mood and a lifting of depression by acting upon the central nervous system. They are powerful in action and should not be taken at the same time as alcohol or other drugs unless under strict medical supervision. Improvement resulting from taking antidepressants may not be noticed for two or three weeks and the patient should be told this. These drugs do have certain unpleasant side effects, such as constipation or diarrhoea, nausea, dry mouth and skin rashes.

One group of drugs, the monoamine oxidase inhibitors (MAOI), cause hypertension if foods such as cheese or Marmite and other antidepressant drugs are taken at the same time.

Tranquillizers. These drugs also act on the central nervous system and exert a calming effect on the patient, but do not make him fall asleep. There are minor tranquillizers which are given to control anxiety and minor fears, but the most important are the major tranquillizers such as chlorpromazine (Largactil) which is given to patients with major illness or disturbance in behaviour.

The side effects of these drugs include postural hypotension, jaundice, skin rashes and changes in muscle tone causing similar effects to the symptoms of Parkinson's disease.

Hypnotics. These are tablets that send a patient to sleep and today very many people use drugs like the barbiturates for this purpose. These may be of some use for a short period of time, but unfortunately it is too easy to become dependent on them and to find them difficult to give up. In general people should be encouraged to try to manage without sleeping tablets as far as possible.

Electroconvulsive therapy (ECT)

In ECT a current of electricity is passed through the cells of the brain under a general anaesthetic, usually to treat depressive illness and a course of six to twelve treatments may be given over a period of three to six weeks.

The nurse has to prepare the patient physically for the treatment by making sure that he does not eat or drink anything for six hours before the anaesthetic. Since treatment is usually given in the morning this means that the patient has no breakfast. Dentures and hair grips are removed, if worn, and the patient, after emptying his bladder is given atropine 0·6 mg as premedication half an hour before the treatment is due to begin. A muscle relaxant may be prescribed. He may be fearful of the treatment, especially the first one and the nurse will need to give him confidence by explaining the procedure and listening to his fears and discussing them with him.

After treatment the nurse must make sure that the patient's airway is clear and observe his pulse and the colour of his skin, while he sleeps on his bed until he has recovered from the anaesthetic. After treatment he may have some loss of memory, causing some confusion about where his bed is, and he may also mislay personal property. The nurse should be aware of this possibility and try to ensure that the patient is observed and supported by her sympathetic presence. If the patient has a headache this will be eased by the prescription of a mild analgesic such as aspirin.

Occupational therapy and industrial therapy

Occupational therapy is carried out by and under the guidance of specially trained occupational therapists whose aim is to help in the diagnosis of illness and, by use of practical, creative, social and intellectual activities, to assist in the assessment and rehabilitation of patients during their stay in hospital. The occupational therapists will be engaged with patients in the wards, in social situations such as visits to shops, or launderettes, and in many activities in occupational therapy departments. These will range from practical tasks such as sewing, woodwork, basketry and painting, to discussions and general knowledge quizzes; from games to organizing and carrying out social activities and dances involving patients, staff and relatives.

The work of the occupational therapist and nurse often overlap and an atmosphere of mutual understanding and respect can contribute enormously in the welfare and recovery of the patient.

Industrial therapy is a form of treatment aimed at assessing the work capability of patients and is also of value in helping patients who may not have worked for some time to get back into regular working habits in the fairly protected atmosphere of the industrial therapy centre, before they return to the hurly-burly of work outside the hospital.

Behaviour therapy

This is a form of treatment usually carried out by psychiatrists or psychologists, although some nurses are now being trained to use these techniques. There are a number of different techniques but they have the common factor of trying to teach the patient to overcome his problems by relearning how to behave in the situations which cause them.

This form of treatment is used with success in patients who have anxiety symptoms, especially if the anxiety is fixed to particular objects (phobic anxiety).

Desensitization is a technique where the patient is taught to relax the muscles of his body and, when he has learned to do this, he is asked to imagine that he is in the situation that he finds alarming, thinking of it for a short time and then relaxing again. This process is repeated continually until the patient is able to confront the alarming situation without being too anxious.

In another form of behaviour therapy the patient who has fears of travelling on buses may go out with a nurse to ride on a bus, and so be able to overcome his fear in the presence of a sympathetic and supportive person.

Nursing Care

The work of the nurse in caring for and treating patients with mental illness is a most rewarding experience, but because of the nature of the problems encountered it does require a degree of understanding of psychiatric conditions and how these may affect the reactions of nurses and patients. This chapter aims at helping the nurse to deal with some of these problems, whether she is working in general or psychiatric wards of a hospital, or in the patient's home.

Teamwork amongst nurses is of vital importance in caring for the mentally sick and this means that the nurses must be able to rely upon each other for support and should communicate freely and frequently about patients' conditions. If nurses are not working well together the level of care given to patients suffers and patients become anxious and are less likely to recover in this atmosphere.

The work of the individual nurse demands that she should understand her role as a nurse from her own point of view and that of the patient and his family. Nurses are usually thought of by patients as people who work in hospital wards caring for physically ill patients and attending to many purely physical needs during illness which the patient would normally carry out for himself. She may wash, feed and dress him if required. To carry out these tasks the nurse wears a special uniform which gives her identity and authority. The nurse herself sees her work as helping sick people, and much of her work consists of doing things for patients and to patients, which frequently involves close physical contact and care. In many ways the patient is dependent upon the nurse and is usually very grateful for her kindness. In her turn the nurse gains satisfaction from what she does for the patient, from his gratitude and his recovery.

Working with the mentally ill patient presents some differences for both patients and nurses. Firstly most patients with such illnesses do not need to stay in bed and they are usually up and dressed and may not seem to be 'ill' at all. The nurses also may not wear uniform—there are increasing numbers of psychiatric wards where this is so—and this often helps the care of the patients since a potential barrier may be removed and many patients can talk more easily to nurses who are not wearing the usual uniform.

The main difference in relationship between patients and nurses in psychiatric illness is that the nurse is striving to help the patient to regain his independence of thought and action. This may mean at times that the nurse must refrain from giving advice and solutions to patients' problems, even when the patient may seek to put responsibility onto the nurse for his actions and decisions. For the nurse who is used to doing everything for her patients this may sometimes be difficult.

The nurses in the ward provide the basic security and consistency in the environment that makes the patient able to confront his illness in an understanding and safe atmosphere, thus allowing him to get well more quickly. To achieve this nurses need to be consistent in their approach to patients and also honest with them. This helps to create safe boundaries for the patients and gives them confidence in the nursing staff.

Talking and listening

One of the first things often asked by nurses caring for psychiatric patients for the first time is, 'What should I say to them?' There is no simple short answer to this question. There are however certain facts to be kept in mind. The most important function of the nurse is not to talk but to *listen*. Secondly, there are no magic answers to what patients say or ask and thirdly, it is most unlikely that anything a nurse does say will do any great harm to a patient.

Listening to patients is often of great value because many patients are able to unburden themselves of great misery simply by talking to a sympathetic listener and frequently these days people are too busy to find time to listen to each other. It may well be that in listening to a patient the nurse has only occasionally to encourage him to continue with a nod, a smile or a few words, to enable a whole story to emerge. Patients often report that after such a talk their problems seemed easier to deal with, or depression was eased, or solutions appeared.

As well as listening to patients it is often found, if a patient finds difficulty in speaking, that just staying with him in silence can be a comforting gesture which is often appreciated later.

A moment's thought will make it abundantly clear to a nurse that there are no immediate solutions to patients' problems. Nurses are often afraid that they may harm patients by what they say, but it is most unlikely that any one isolated statement can do real harm to a patient, assuming that the nurse does not mean to hurt him.

Involvement with patients

Nurses must be involved with their patients to a certain extent in order to be able to understand and thus help them. However some degree of objectivity and control is desirable for both the patient and the nurse. Recognition of when involvement is not of value to the patient can be made by observing certain developments in the attitudes of the people concerned. When the relationship between a nurse and a patient is carried outside the ward and working hours, when other people are excluded by them, when the nurse feels that she alone understands the patient and when she is unable to discuss the patient freely with her colleagues, the situation has become one which is unlikely to help the patient's treatment. These guidelines should be of use in enabling nurses to be effectively involved with their patients.

Aggression and hostility

These are subjects that can cause anxiety and fear in nurses when they begin to look after psychiatric patients, so some understanding of the basis of these reactions may help the nurse to meet the situation.

Aggression can take either physical or verbal form and both can be upsetting to the nurse unless it is realised that often this behaviour is part of the patient's illness and is not always directed personally at the individual nurse. Patients who are feeling persecuted or have delusions or hallucinations may attack if alarmed or even without any apparent provocation, and it is useful to know how to respond to this or how to avoid situations building up and exploding. If a patient is restless or overactive and tense, efforts can be made to get him to channel this energy in a constructive way, such as a walk or a game of table tennis. Where physical aggression does break out the situation must be dealt with effectively by a number of nurses. A single nurse should never attempt to restrain a patient alone. This might result in a struggle or fight in which someone may get hurt. To restrain a patient at least three and preferably four nurses should co-operate and hold the patient closely and firmly, so that neither the patient nor the nurses gets hurt. This firm holding and control may be comforting to patients who are feeling very frightened.

Delusions and hallucinations

Patients who are deluded or suffering hallucinations may give problems to nurses about the way to respond and treat them. Nurses should not attempt to argue with patients about delusions or hallucinations, nor is there any need to agree with them. The most appropriate course of action, usually, is to try to distract the patient from the topic by involving him in some other point of conversation, or diverting him into some activity.

Feeding patients

Feeding those with psychiatric illness is a cause of conflict at times, and some patients require all a nurse's skill and ingenuity to ensure that they take an adequate diet. Patients who are depressed may refuse to eat because they believe that because of their unworthiness they have no right to food, or that their bowels are blocked so that food cannot pass through. Other patients may refuse food believing it to be poisoned. Patients who are overactive may not sit down long enough to eat meals, but will often eat snacks or sandwiches if offered. For patients who refuse food the nurse must ensure that at least some fluids are taken. Often a patient can be persuaded to have a drink, but the nurse must stay by him to make sure that it is taken. It may take an hour to get a patient to take a glass of milk! Oral hygiene is particularly important in patients who refuse food and the nurse has a responsibility to see that this is properly carried out.

Sleep

Sleep is often disturbed for psychiatric patients and the night nurse can often be a comfort to those who have difficulty in sleeping. Darkness may make the night a long and frightening time if a patient cannot sleep and the nurse should not automatically reach for the bottle of sleeping tablets, since the sleep that they give is not entirely satisfactory. Patients may be able to sleep after talking to the nurse and she should provide a listening ear and also comfort in the form of a cup of tea, coffee or milk to help him gain a few precious hours of natural sleep. Those who do not sleep at night but have catnaps during the day should be encouraged to stay awake during the day so that they are more likely to sleep at night.

Suicide

This is something that a nurse is certain to meet during the course of her training and the patients she cares for will include those who have tried to kill themselves. In caring for a patient who has taken an overdose of tablets or injured himself in a suicidal attempt, physical care will be needed to rid the body of poisons or repair any other damage.

Care of the patient after recovery from the poisoning or injuries is of the greatest importance to prevent further attempts and to help the patient back to health.

People who attempt suicide may be making a cry for help or expressing their despair with life, and to be of help the nurse must have a sympathetic and understanding manner. The patient will often feel guilty about his attempt and the nurse should not make the burden of guilt heavier by reproaching him and expressing anger or hostility towards him, nor should she ignore him or tell him 'to pull himself together'. Most people who do kill themselves have usually given a hint of their intentions and this is something that a nurse should be looking and listening for, especially in patients who are depressed.

The work of the nurse in caring for patients with psychiatric illness can thus be described as providing a stable, secure environment where the needs of the patient as a person can be met. The nurse is alert to the physical needs of the patients, and observes their social behaviour towards each other and with the nurses. She provides sympathetic support and comfort to enable her patients to function independently once again. She must learn to observe and report on the behaviour of patients both verbally and in writing to her colleagues, since these observations are of great value in assessing the patient's progress and response to treatment.

The Future

During the last decade a different approach to the care of the patient with mental illness has developed and there is a trend away from hospital care. The number of hospital beds is falling and many patients are admitted to hospital for short periods only, many now going to the psychiatric units in District General Hospitals where they can be closer to their home surroundings. Day hospitals have been established in many areas where patients attend during the day, and go home in the evenings and at the week-ends.

The patient's family is encouraged to take part in his care, with the help and support of psychiatric nurses working in the community who treat patients in their own homes. For example Dingleton Hospital in Scotland has close links with the local community and many patients are treated at home by the hospital staff in conjunction with the general practitioners.

Local Authorities have an important part to play in community treatment since they provide many facilities and help with assessment and rehabilitation of patients. In the reorganized National Health Service which came into force in 1974 hospital and community care are much more closely linked, and there is also close liaison with the services provided by Local Government leading, it is hoped, to a more efficient and effective treatment of patients.

9

The Nurse and the Hospital

The Nurse and Her Patient

When someone is ill he may experience pain and discomfort, and at least become generally aware that something is wrong. When he is admitted to hospital there is also a marked change in his daily routine and surroundings and this, together with his symptoms, continually remind him that he is now a patient. It is one of your prime tasks to make him feel that he is still a person.

The sheer courage and determination of many patients to overcome their illness and pain will astonish you. But the attitudes and behaviour of others range from the petulantly childish and whining to the overbearingly rude and demanding; some are weak, timid and anxious to please while others lose no opportunity to grumble. The common factor is fear—fear of the unknown ward and the unknown people and fear of the unforseeable future.

In everyday life there are many different sorts of relationship; husband and wife or brother and sister are equals but teacher and pupil or parent and child clearly are not. However, some relationships are more subtle. The brilliantly clever lawyer or the rich pop star who takes his car to be repaired, quite happily accepts the diagnosis and treatment recommended by the garage mechanic!

As soon as you put on your uniform, and however junior you may be, you as a nurse assume responsibility for your patients' care; you watch carefully to see what progress they make and report what you see to the ward sister or doctor. But remember that you too are being watched by your patients from the moment you first meet. So you greet the new arrival pleasantly and politely and immediately set about making him feel that he is going to be looked after very carefully and efficiently.

A person who is ill or in pain is very often confused and will appreciate a quiet and gentle introduction to life in hospital. Make a note of his worries and see that sister hears about them. Soothing words have a valuable place in medicine but your patient will soon lose faith in you if he finds that his anxieties about home, family and pets are not resolved; the social services are there to be used.

Many of your nursing procedures are ones which in other circumstances would be very embarrassing to you and your patient and which even in hospital may still embarrass the patient. So be polite, discreet and matter-of-fact. Be friendly but not familiar or saucy or you will find yourself being treated casually too.

Your patient's attitude to you depends not only on your attitude to him but on your sheer nursing skill. Be sure that there are no painful injections or dropped instruments, no bed sores nor slipping dressings caused by your negligence. In fact be and always look professional and take a pride in your appearance. Your own confidence will communicate itself to the ward and serve to remind people that you are a person on whom they can rely.

Admission of a Patient to Hospital

A patient may be admitted from the consultant's waiting list or as an emergency admission. In most hospitals he is admitted to the ward via reception. He may be accompanied by relatives or friends who should be asked to wait in the waiting room while preliminary details are taken down and admission forms filled in and an identity bracelet put on. The patient and his relatives are then taken to the ward by a member of the reception area staff or by a nurse.

On arrival in the ward the nurse admitting the patient introduces herself by name to the patient and his relatives with a pleasant, smiling manner. A smile is one of the quickest and happiest ways of reassuring people. If he is well enough she then escorts the patient to the dayroom or part of the ward reserved for the reception of new patients, the relatives staying with him. By greeting the patient in this way she can reassure him and make him feel expected.

If the patient is very ill on admission, he is brought from the reception area on a trolley and put straight into bed, lying if necessary on a blanket in which he can be wrapped for undressing. The bed should have been prepared for his reception and any equipment, such as extra pillows and backrest put ready beside it.

In some hospitals special 'admission' forms are filled in in the ward by the ward clerk and to complete them the following information is usually required:

(1) Date of admission.
(2) Name and address of the patient.
(3) Whether married or single.
(4) Name and address of general practitioner.
(5) Name of physician or surgeon in charge of the patient.
(6) Name, address and telephone number of next of kin.
(7) Religion (optional).
(8) Age of patient.
(9) Occupation.

If the patient's next of kin is not on the telephone it is important to get the name, address and telephone number of a relative, friend or neighbour who would be willing to take a message or, failing that, the address and telephone number of the nearest police station.

Relatives should be given any other information that they will need. Most hospitals issue a booklet giving times of visiting and any other information. If a patient is likely to need an operation his consent must be obtained, or in the case of a child under sixteen the consent of his parents but it is wise to obtain the consent of the parent or guardian if possible for a person between the ages of sixteen and eighteen years of age. The responsibility for obtaining consent rests with the doctor.

After this the patient can be shown to his bed and the relatives given the opportunity before leaving the ward of seeing him settled and to say goodbye. This also gives them the chance to see where his bed is situated so that they can visualize him in his new surroundings. They should also see the nurse in charge of the ward before leaving.

After the relatives have gone the patient may be introduced to the other patients and, if he is able to walk, shown the general layout of the ward, including the bathroom and lavatory. This helps him to feel more at home. He is encouraged to put photographs and other personal possessions on his locker to remind him of home. He should be given a brief outline of the ward routine, including mealtimes, times of the doctors' rounds and the times when the staff change duty and anything else that seems to be important to make him feel more at ease.

Preliminary observations and assessment of the patient should be made, noting his general condition and symptoms. His temperature, pulse and respirations are recorded and a specimen of urine collected for testing. Many hospitals bath the patient at this point and weigh him if his condition permits. Others leave it until the normal bathing time to allow him a little more time to get used to his surroundings. While bathing him the nurse should take this opportunity of noting and reporting any sores, bruises, rashes and other abnormalities.

Toilet requisites such as flannels, soap, toothbrush, brush and comb, as well as night attire, dressing-gown and slippers, are usually provided by the patient but if he has not got them they can be given from the ward stores.

Patients should be advised to hand over any money and valuables for safe keeping. It is better that he keeps only the minimum of possessions with him in hospital but if the family cannot take his clothes and valuables home with them the nurse should obtain instructions about them from the nurse in charge of the ward, as rulings on this vary from hospital to hospital. Enquiry should also be made about any drugs he may have in his possession and these should be collected and handed in for the duration of his stay.

The nurse should leave the patient comfortable in readiness for the doctor's visit and report all the observations made during the admission procedure to the nurse in charge.

10

Care of the Patient in Bed

Bed-making is one of the first things that a new nurse learns to do and it is one of the most important of her nursing duties. Patients spend most of their stay in hospital in bed and their comfort, rest and sleep depend on the skill and efficiency of their nurses.

Bed-making is usually done by two nurses working together. If the patient is well enough to get up, he can be sat in a chair, wearing a dressing-gown and away from a draught. This is a good time to chat with your patients and to get to know them. Keep a watchful eye on the patient in case the effort of sitting up is too much for him. When you have finished making the bed, always ask if the patient is comfortable before leaving him. See that his head is properly supported, that the clothes are not tight over his chest and that his locker is by his side with everything within reach.

To make a bed

If the patient is lying down. If the patient cannot get out of bed, the bed is made around him while he lies down. The procedure is as follows:

(1) Two chairs are placed back to back at the foot of the bed so that the bedclothes can be placed on them.

(2) Starting at the head of the bed, untuck the bedclothes down to the foot.

(3) Remove each article separately, folding it loosely and hanging it over the backs of the other two chairs, making sure that the ends do not trail on the floor.

(4) Leave the last blanket on as a cover for the patient and remove the top sheet by drawing it down towards the foot of the bed, underneath the blanket.

(5) Pull the mattress back into position if, as often happens, it has slipped towards the foot of the bed.

(6) On the side of the bed which had the least amount of drawsheet tucked in:

The nurse on this side leans over the patient (keeping him covered with the blanket), places one hand under his shoulders and the other under his hips, and gently rolls him over towards her. She supports him in this position while the other nurse moves the pillow so that his head is resting comfortably.

(7) Straighten the underblanket and sheet, brushing out any crumbs and tuck them both back firmly.

(8) Tuck in about 30 cm (12 in) of the drawsheet and gather the rest in a roll against the patient's back.

(9) Roll the patient gently back and over on to the other side.

(10) Brush and straighten out the sheet and underblanket on the other side and tuck them in.

(11) Unroll the drawsheet, brush it free of crumbs and tuck it in firmly, folding the extra length under the mattress, so that the patient has a cool, fresh portion on which to lie.

(12) Roll him gently on to his back again and arrange his pillows comfortably.

(13) Spread the top sheet over the bed and withdraw the blanket from underneath it.

(14) Tuck the sheet in at the bottom, making a generous pleat over his feet so that he can move them without restriction.

If the patient is sitting up. Some patients, for example those suffering from breathlessness, spend most of their time in bed sitting upright. The bed-making procedure is then varied as follows:

(1) Strip the top bedclothes, leaving one blanket covering the patient.

(2) Untuck the bottom sheet, lift the patient's feet, straighten the underblanket and tuck the sheet in again firmly.

(3) Keeping the patient well-covered, lift him down to the bottom of the bed. One nurse now supports him while the other remakes the top of the bed.

(4) Lift the patient back to his original position and finish the rest of the bed.

(5) If the patient cannot be moved in this way two nurses must then lift him where he is while a third straightens the underblanket, tucks the sheet in and pulls the drawsheet through.

To change the bottom sheet

If the patient is lying down. The procedure is as follows:

(1) Strip the top of the bed, keeping the patient covered with a blanket.

(2) Untuck the bottom sheet.

(3) Roll the clean sheet up lengthwise until it is only half its width.

(4) Gently roll the patient over onto one side.

(5) Roll the bottom sheet up against the patient's back together with the drawsheet.

(6) Place the clean sheet in position, tucking it firmly in and with the rolled side up against the patient's back. Tuck in the drawsheet in the same way.

(7) Roll the patient over the sheets and onto his other side.

(8) Take out the soiled sheet, unroll the clean one and complete the bed in the usual way.

If the patient is sitting up. The procedure is as follows:

(1) Strip the bed in the usual way, leaving the patient covered by a blanket.

(2) Untuck the bottom sheet.

(3) Move the patient to the bottom of the bed.

(4) Roll the clean sheet along the width and put it in from the top of the bed, rolling back the soiled sheet.

(5) Lift the patient back into position, over the two rolled sheets. Be careful to keep the patient covered and supported all the time.

(6) Remove the soiled sheet and tuck the clean sheet firmly into position.

Soiled linen

After bed-making, used linen is placed in the used linen container, sealed and sent to the laundry. Soiled linen which is linen soiled with blood, urine or faeces is placed in a plastic bag, for the protection of the laundry staff, sealed and sent to the laundry without delay. The linen contains micro-organisms and should never be shaken about or handled more than absolutely necessary in the ward. Nurses must always wash their hands after handling it.

Aids to comfort in bed

Hot water-bottles. Because of the risk of burning the patient hot water-bottles are not often used, and should only be used with the permission of the sister in charge of the ward. They should never be used for the unconscious or anaesthetized patient, nor for anyone with any loss of sensation or paralysis. When filling them, make sure that all air is expelled from the bottle, that the cap is screwed on very securely and that they are completely encased in a thick cover.

Electric pads and blankets should be used with the same care for the patient's safety, owing to the risk of burning and also to the risk of electric shock if the bed becomes wet. They are mainly used to warm the bed when it is unoccupied and are removed when the bed is in use.

Backrests are usually incorporated into the framework of the bed-head and can be adjusted to various angles.

Bed cradles are metal frames used to take the weight of the bedding from the patient or to prevent the bedding interfering with splints and other appliances. They are used whenever they can add to the patient's comfort and are also used to promote free circulation of air around plaster of Paris when it is drying.

Rubber or foam-plastic rings are used to relieve pressure on the sacral area of the body and are enclosed in a cotton cover. Ripple beds and sheepskins can be used for the same reason. After use they must be disinfected and stored flat in a dark cupboard.

Pulleys. By means of a pulley attached to the top of the bed a patient may help himself up in bed to relieve pressure on his sacrum.

Positions used in Nursing

The position adopted for nursing a patient often depends on the disease from which he is suffering and the resulting symptoms. When a patient is nursed in any of these positions the nurse must see that he is supported comfortably and that the position is maintained.

The recumbent position

The patient lies on his back with his head on one or two pillows and legs either straight or slightly flexed. This may be used:

(1) When complete relaxation is required in acute illness, e.g. rheumatic fever.

(2) Occasionally for a patient suffering from shock, e.g. after an operation.

(3) After some spinal anaesthetics.

The semi-recumbent position allows the patient to see about him and also ensures that he will not fall forward.

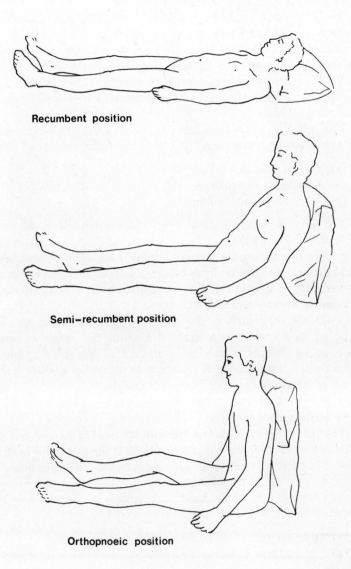

Recumbent position

Semi-recumbent position

Orthopnoeic position

Fig. 1. Three dorsal nursing positions.

The orthopnoeic and upright positions

The orthopnoeic position is sometimes used for patients suffering from advanced heart failure who have difficulty in breathing. The patient is supported sitting upright with a backrest and several pillows. In addition, a 'heart table' may be improvised by placing a pillow on the top of the bed table in front of the patient so that he can lean forwards on it if he wishes. Alternatively, a Lawson-Tait cardiac bed may be used.

The upright position is when the patient's trunk is raised so that he is in a sitting position and may be achieved by the use of either:

(1) Several pillows.
(2) A backrest and pillows.
(3) A Lawson–Tait–Fowler bed.

The latter includes a knee support, which also prevents the patient from slipping down the bed. In the absence of this, a foot rest of some sort will prevent the patient from slipping down. This position allows fluid in the abdominal cavity to collect in the pelvic region rather than beneath the diaphragm and so consequently it is used after some abdominal operations and in inflammation of abdominal organs, e.g. appendicitis, peritonitis. It also prevents the abdominal organs from pressing on the diaphragm and thus allowing the patient to breathe more easily. It is often used after abdominal operations to prevent chest complications and is of great help to patients with disease of the heart or lungs who have difficulty in breathing.

The semi-prone position

The patient lies face downward with his head turned on one side. Pillows are placed under his chest and under the side of his head and face. The patient usually places his arms, flexed, on either side of his head or any other comfortable position. Another small pillow is usually required under the front of the ankles, to keep his toes from pressing on the bed. This is used when required for:

(1) Drainage from abdominal and chest wounds.
(2) For a patient suffering from wounds, burns or other injuries of the back.
(3) As an alternative position to relieve pressure on other parts of the body when a patient is confined to bed for a long time.
(4) For the relief of flatulence.

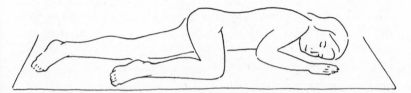

Fig. 2. The semi-prone position.

The left lateral position

In this position the patient is nursed on one side, with one to three pillows placed comfortably under the head. Sometimes the back is supported by another pillow. The knee may be flexed. In quite helpless patients a pillow may be placed between the knees to avoid pressure. This is used as an alternative to the dorsal recumbent

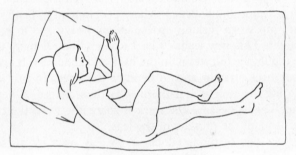

Left lateral position

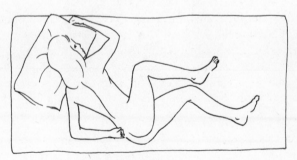

Sims's position

Fig. 3. Positions used for rectal and vaginal examinations; the left lateral gives complete relaxation to the resting patient.

position for complete relaxation and to relieve pressure on the back. The left lateral position may also be used when carrying out treatments, for example preparing a patient for rectal examination or giving an enema. For this the buttocks are brought to the edge of the bed with thighs and knees flexed.

Sims's position

This position is sometimes used for examination of the vagina. The patient lies on her left side with her chest in the semi-prone position, her left side and leg near to the side of the bed, her left arm behind her back, her right knee drawn up so that the heel touches the left knee and her right arm is extended forwards.

Lifting Patients

It is most important that a nurse should learn to lift patients, both for her own sake and the patient's. Many people tend to bend from the waist and hip when picking up something heavy and to keep their legs straight. This way leads to backache and occasionally to hernia because it puts the full strain on the back and abdomen. It is better to keep your back straight and to bend at the knee. In this way it is easier to lift the weight and there is far less chance of developing backache. This is because the work is shared between the back, the abdomen and all the muscles of the legs.

There are two methods which are widely used by nurses when lifting patients, the arm lift and the shoulder lift. The essence of each of them is to *keep your back straight* and *bend your knees*.

11

Observing and Reporting

Temperature

The patient should be nursed at a temperature which is comfortable in relation to his condition, i.e. 18°C (65°F) unless the doctor orders it to be higher for children, old people, or people suffering from diseases of the lungs or chest.

A thermometer is an instrument used to record temperatures. A clinical thermometer, used for taking the temperature of the body, consists of a narrow glass tube with a bulb containing mercury and a stem through the centre of which runs a tiny hollow tube. Divisions or degrees from 35 to 43°C (95 to 110°F) are marked on the stem by black lines so that the height of the mercury is easily seen. The space between each degree is divided into ten smaller spaces. On a Fahrenheit thermometer the space between degrees is divided into five smaller spaces each representing two-tenths. As the mercury in the tube becomes heated, it expands and rises up the tube and can be seen as a thin silver thread. A rectal thermometer has a special thick rounded bulb. There is also a universal type which can be used for any method but if used rectally must be very clearly marked and kept for this purpose. The normal temperature of the body is 36–37°C (97–99°F), and varies very little in health.

Unless a patient is very ill, when his temperature is recorded four-hourly or more often, it is taken morning and evening, though this practice is often discontinued after the temperature has been normal for some days unless the patient develops fresh symptoms.

Celsius and Fahrenheit

Two scales of temperature are in common use, Celsius and Fahrenheit. *Note:* Celsius is the new name for what has for a long time been called the Centigrade scale; the abbreviation is still °C.

You need remember only three temperatures on each scale and these are:

Boiling point of water	100°C	212°F
Normal blood temperature (approx.)	37°C	98·6°F
Freezing point of water	0°C	32°F

It may occasionally be necessary to convert degrees Fahrenheit to degrees Celsius or Celsius to Fahrenheit; the easiest method to *remember* is based on the fact that −40°C is the same temperature as −40°F.

To convert Fahrenheit to Celsius
Example: convert 212°F to °C:

Method	Example
1. Add 40	$212 + 40 = 252$
2. Multiply by 5	$252 \times 5 = 1260$
3. Divide by 9	$1260 \div 9 = 140$
4. Subtract 40	$140 - 40 = 100°C$

To convert Celsius to Fahrenheit
Example: convert 37°C to °F:

Method	Example
1. Add 40	$37 + 40 = 77$
2. Multiply by 9	$77 \times 9 = 693$
3. Divide by 5	$693 \div 5 = 138·6$
4. Subtract 40	$138·6 - 40 = 98·6°F$

To help you to remember:
In both conversions steps 1 and 4 are the same.
Fahrenheit is a bigger word than Celsius and degrees Fahrenheit is always a bigger number than degrees Celsius.

How to take the temperature

The temperature of the body may be taken in the mouth, in the axilla or groin or in the rectum. A nurse must always insert and remove a thermometer herself. She must thoroughly rinse, clean and disinfect it after use and hold it in position in the case of children, restless patients and those who are unconscious or delirious.
Requirements. These are as follows:

Jar containing a thermometer.

Bowl of cold water free from disinfectant for rinsing the thermometer.

Swabs for drying the thermometer.

Receiver for swabs.

The temperature is recorded as a graph on a special chart ruled for the purpose. This must be kept very accurately and neatly.

Procedure. The procedure is as follows:

In the mouth. Do not give either a hot or a cold drink immediately before taking the temperature by this method. Wipe the thermometer. See that the mercury has been shaken down to below 35°C (95°F). Place the bulb under the tongue and close the lips, telling the patient to be careful not to bite the thermometer. It should be left in place for two minutes. *Never* take the temperature in the mouth either of young children or of patients who are delirious, unconscious or who have difficulty in breathing.

In the axilla, i.e. under the arm. Wipe the axilla with a swab. Place the thermometer in position and see that it is not in contact with any clothing or with a hot water-bottle. Draw the patient's arm across the chest. Leave for at least three minutes.

This method should not be used immediately after the patient has had a hot bath.

In the rectum. This method is useful in the case of infants and after accidents in the case of adults when it is not possible to use any other method. A rectal thermometer should always be kept in a specially marked container and should be greased before it is inserted. It is left in place for one minute.

The temperature in the rectum is half a degree higher than in the mouth and in the mouth it is half a degree higher than in the axilla or groin.

All thermometers should be left in position for at least twice as long as the time stated on them. The interval is used for counting the pulse and respirations.

In cases where an unexpected temperature reading occurs, the nurse should retake it with another thermometer.

Immediately after use, hold the thermometer firmly between the thumb and first finger of the right hand and flick from the wrist to shake the mercury down. Then wash it in cold water, wipe it and place it bulb downwards in a glass jar containing suitable disinfectant. The bulb should be protected by a swab of cotton wool placed in the bottom of the jar. Each patient should have a separate thermo-meter.

Terms used in connection with an abnormal temperature

A *subnormal* temperature is one below 36°C (96·8°F). This occurs when the blood pressure is very low, as in shock or after severe bleeding, or near death, when a person has been subjected to severe cold over a long period, especially if this is accompanied by mal-nutrition and when a patient's temperature is deliberately reduced to 30°C (86°F), or even lower, during operations (hypothermia). *Pyrexia* is fever, i.e. a temperature over 37·2°B (99°F) rising to about 40°C (104°F). *Hyperpyrexia*, higher still, is very rare except in malaria, or occasionally before death from some brain disease.

Rigor

A rigor is an acute attack of shivering which may occur at the onset, or during the course of, an acute infection like pneumonia or menin-gitis. It has three stages:

(1) The cold stage, in which the patient is blue, cold and shivering.

(2) The hot stage, in which the patient is flushed, with dry skin, severe headache, full bounding pulse and rising temperature.

(3) The sweating stage, in which there is profuse perspiration, the temperature falls rapidly and usually the pulse and general condition improve.

A rigor is always very serious and must be reported at once.

Shivering without a rise of temperature or sweating may be due to cold, fatigue or emotion.

Treatment. When a rigor commences the nurse should place a warm blanket next to the patient. More blankets may be piled on the bed until the shivering stops. The temperature should be taken in the axilla.

When the hot stage is reached the blankets should be removed and a cold drink given. A cold compress may be placed on the forehead. During this stage the temperature is recorded every fifteen minutes. If it rises above 40·5°C (105°F) tepid sponging may be ordered. The temperature should be taken again to note the limit the pyrexia has reached.

When the patient begins to sweat, sponge him down with warm water taking care not to chill him and change his clothing as often as may be necessary. The rigor may well exhaust the patient and his colour and pulse must be carefully watched. If a stimulant has been ordered it may be given at the end of the rigor and if the patient is then made comfortable he may sleep. During the course of a rigor the patient is never left alone. The temperatures should be charted in red ink and the word 'Rigor' added.

Sponging

Sponging is a measure which may be undertaken to reduce the temperature of the body in fever by approximately 1°C and for its soothing effect on the patient. It has a cooling effect because it increases the amount of evaporation of moisture from the surface of the body, therefore the skin should be left damp.

Requirements for tepid sponging. These are as follows:

Clean, warm clothing.
The patient's own bath blanket.
Clinical thermometer.
Large washing bowl.
Water at 32°C (90°F), which may be allowed to cool to 24°C (75°F).
Bath thermometer.
Two jugs, one of hot and one of cold water.
Pail for change of water.
Five sponges.
Bowl to receive surplus water from sponge.
Small bowl of iced water with compress for the forehead.
Ice cubes in bowl.
The patient's brush and comb.

Procedure. The procedure is as follows:

(1) Place screens round the bed and close the windows to ensure privacy and prevent draughts.

(2) Gently roll one bath blanket under the patient and cover him with another.

(3) Soak, squeeze lightly and place a cold sponge in each axilla and on each groin.

(4) Sponge and dry the face and, if the temperature is very high, place a cold compress on the forehead.

(5) Using the sponges alternately and with long sweeping strokes sponge the arms in turn, then the body and legs.

(6) Do not dry the skin, but leave it damp in order to allow cooling of the surfaces by evaporation.

(7) Take the temperature and compare it with that taken before the sponging. Stop treatment when it has fallen 1°C.

(8) Wait until the skin is dry.

(9) Remove the bottom blanket, straightening the bottom sheet and drawsheet.

(10) Put clean pyjamas on the patient.

(11) Brush and comb the hair with as little disturbance as possible.

(12) Remove the upper bath blanket and cover with a sheet and a blanket.

(13) Give a suitable drink, e.g. lemonade and take the temperature again, half an hour later.

(14) The procedure should take about twenty minutes and care should be taken to move the patient as little as possible.

The Pulse

A good indication of a patient's condition is the wave of movement which passes along the wall of an artery every time the heart beats. It is felt wherever an artery passes over a bone fairly near the skin. The radial artery in the wrist is the best example of this.

How to count the pulse

Lay the patient's arm on the bed with the elbow and wrist slightly flexed and place three fingers on the hollow so formed over the artery. Do not count the pulse immediately after exertion; let the patient settle down and then start counting. In the case of nervous patients, keep on counting for a longer period than the usual time of one minute.

A nurse must notice the frequency, quality and regularity of the pulse. By frequency is meant the number of beats in a given time. This should be about one hundred and twenty per minute in the case of a small child, seventy two per minute in the case of an adult and sixty per minute in the case of an old person. By quality is meant the strength of the pulse, e.g. full and bounding in some forms of heart disease, thin and thready in collapse and haemorrhage.

A pulse is said to be: (*a*) *regular* when the beats are equal in strength and when the pause between them is always of the same length; (*b*) *irregular* when the beats vary in force and rhythm. This occurs in some forms of serious heart disease; (*c*) *intermittent* when there is an occasional dropped beat; and (*d*) *running* when the beats are so rapid that they cannot be counted; this may occur after prolonged bleeding.

A nurse must always report any abnormal pulse to the sister or nurse in charge of the ward especially when she is keeping a quarter-hourly pulse chart after accident or operation. A rising pulse rate may be the only indication of internal haemorrhage and the nurse taking it may be the only one to know until it is too late. She must report it at once if the pulse rate is higher than the last time she took it. As a general rule, the weaker the pulse, the more dangerous the condition of the patient, while a falling temperature with an increase in the pulse rate is a very serious sign. A slowing pulse can indicate increasing head injury and this must be reported.

Respiration

The normal respiration rate is between sixteen and twenty breaths a minute and should be counted when the patient is unaware that this is being done, by keeping the fingers on the wrist as though still counting the pulse. A nurse should notice whether the respirations are quick, noisy or quiet, shallow or deep, difficult or easy, regular or irregular. Breathing should be quiet and deep, but in some diseases it alters to rest the affected part. It is shallow in cases of shock, collapse, peritonitis and pleurisy, it is quicker in children, in feverish conditions and as a result of emotion and exertion; it is slower in brain disease and head injury; and it is noisy in chest disease and stroke.

The term *dyspnoea* means difficult breathing. Sighing is a sign that the body is not receiving a sufficient amount of oxygen and occurs in shock and collapse. Cheyne–Stokes breathing is always a very grave sign and can often be heard shortly before death in diseases of vital organs, e.g. heart and brain.

A nurse must draw the attention of the sister or nurse in charge of the ward to any abnormal sounds heard in connection with the patient's breathing.

Apex Beat

The apex beat of the heart is sometimes recorded for comparison with the radial pulse rate. In normal persons the apex of the heart is on a level with the fifth intercostal space, 9 cm (3·5 in) from the midline. In disease it may be considerably displaced to the left. A stethoscope is placed over the apex of the heart and the number of beats per minute is recorded. At the same time the radial pulse is counted for one minute. Two nurses are required to make both these observations simultaneously, one counting the pulse and the other listening to the apex beat through a stethoscope.

Blood Pressure

Blood pressure is usually measured in the brachial artery. This should be done while the patient is at rest, with the arm supported comfortably. If the patient is receiving treatment for high blood pressure, the pressure should first be taken while he is lying down and then after he has stood up one minute. This is in order to record whether there is a fall in blood pressure due to change in posture.

In order to avoid errors due to nervousness on the part of the patient, the room should be as quiet as possible. The patient should not be allowed to get cold because this will affect the reading. If the pulse is rapid this suggests emotional stress and the blood pressure should be repeated after a short period of lying down.

Two readings are taken when recording blood pressure, the systolic (peak pressure) and diastolic (lowest pressure). In a healthy young adult the normal values are 120 and 80 mm of mercury respectively and are written 120/80. The inflatable cuff of a sphygmomanometer is wrapped firmly round the patient's upper arm and the cuff inflated until the pulse at the wrist can no longer be felt. The pressure is increased by a further 10–20 mmHg, the stethoscope placed over the site of the now silent brachial pulse and the sphygmomanometer gradually deflated until the pulse is heard, at which point the pressure is noted (systolic). The cuff is deflated further until the quality of the sound changes and that pressure noted (diastolic).

Writing Reports

The daily nursing record

On admission the patient has an individual card prepared with name, age, date of admission and provisional diagnosis. The nurse in charge writes notes on the patient's condition, nursing treatment required and specific instructions from the medical staff each morning and evening. These day-to-day entries are really comprehensive and should include the following:

(1) An accurate account of any drugs given and their effect on the patient and the time the next dose is due.

(2) The nature of any dressings carried out, e.g. removal of stitches, renewals of dressings, repacking of wounds.

(3) The nature of any patient's pain and steps taken to relieve it.

(4) The time and nature of any vomiting and its relationship to food.

(5) The quantity and nature of nourishment taken especially fluids.

(6) Bowel and bladder action and, when necessary, the amount of urine passed.

(7) Whether specimens have been sent to the laboratory.

(8) The patient's mental state.

(9) How much rest the patient has had.

Any other information of importance to the sister or doctor should also be noted down.

The day sister's report

This report is written by the sister or nurse in charge of the ward for the information of the senior administrative nursing staff and the night sisters. The report will include details of the following:

(1) New patients.

(2) Patients prepared for operations.

(3) Postoperative patients.

(4) Patients who have had special investigations or treatments.

(5) Incidents such as injury sustained by a patient in a fall or the names of patients who have been discharged irregularly.

(6) Seriously ill patients.

(7) Patients who have died.

Night nurse's report

This report is normally written for each ward by the nurse in charge at night. It covers the twenty-four hour period.

The twenty-four hour report

The day sister's and the night nurse's report are often combined in one twenty-four hour report.

12

Storage and Administration of Drugs

A drug is any substance or mixture of substances administered to patients in the treatment or prevention of disease. Preparations of such drugs are usually known as medicine. Those which contain poisons, dangerous or habit-forming substances are controlled in the United Kingdom by the Misuse of Drugs Act 1973 and other Poison Acts and Pharmacy Acts.

Storage of Drugs

All drugs should be kept locked up in clearly labelled cupboards away from patients. Those controlled by the Misuse of Drugs Act and Pharmacy Acts must be locked securely in special cupboards and only the trained nurse in charge of the ward keeps the key. Lotions for external application may also be in a locked cupboard but kept separate from drugs to be taken internally. This security is necessary because drug dependency will often lead to very serious physical, mental and social effects for the individual concerned.

Controlled drugs in common use are cocaine, morphine, papaveretum, pethidine, amphetamines, methaqualone (including Mandrax), phenoperidine, dextromoramide, diamorphine, methadone, and dihydrocodeine.

All these controlled drugs are labelled 'C.D.' and must be stored separately in a locked cupboard to be labelled Controlled Drugs; this must be within another locked cupboard. Some hospitals use specially designed drug trolleys, padlocked to the wall when not in use. Keys must be kept on the person of the sister or charge nurse or deputy all the time. The keys must all be kept on the same keyring and should not be relinquished to anyone else, apart from the ward pharmacist when he inspects the trolley or cupboard.

Schedule 1 poisons

Those drugs labelled 'S.1.' and other drugs that the nursing and pharmacy staff have agreed should be treated in the same way are labelled in red print on a white ground, with the additional phrase 'Store in Poisons Cupboard'. This cupboard is labelled S.1. The key to this cupboard is on the same keyring as the C.D. key and is therefore subject to the same safeguards.

All drugs not labelled C.D. or 'store in poisons cupboard'

Preparations for internal use with the exception of fluid for intravenous infusion and for irrigation must be stored in a locked cupboard. Antibiotics and other therapeutic substances may require storage in a refrigerator.

Preparations for external use may be stored in unlocked cupboards provided that supervision of patients is adequate; circumstances will vary in different departments. All preparations in psychiatric wards must be kept in a locked cupboard when not in use.

Urine testing reagents should be kept in a locked cupboard, the key being kept in a safe place accessible to the nursing staff.

Administration of Drugs

Drugs can be administered in many forms, i.e. as capsules, emulsions, injections, mixtures, ointments, powders, suppositories, drops and tablets. They are given:

(1) By mouth, to be swallowed or dissolved under the tongue.
(2) By injection.
(3) By topical application, i.e. to the skin.
(4) By inhalation.
(5) By rectum, in suppositories or enemas.

Many abbreviations are unfortunately still used by older doctors in writing prescriptions but a nurse is perfectly entitled to ask for clarification.

Measuring drugs

Today metric measurements are universally used for drugs. Measurements required in drug dosage are:

Volume. The unit of measure is the litre (l). Each litre contains 1000 millilitres (ml). The cubic centimetre (cc) is occasionally used instead of the millilitre. They are, however, almost exactly equal, but the cc is now an obsolete unit.

Weight. The unit of measure is the kilogramme (kg). Each kilogramme contains 1000 grams (g). Each gram contains 1000 milligrams (mg). Each milligram contains 1000 micrograms. The abbreviation for microgram is μg but this should always be written in full as it is easily mistaken for mg.

The decimal point: There are no fractions in the metric system. Instead the decimal point is used:

$$0\cdot1 = 1/10 \qquad 0\cdot5 = 5/10 \quad = \tfrac{1}{2}$$
$$0\cdot01 = 1/100 \qquad 0\cdot05 = 5/100 \quad = 1/20$$
$$0\cdot001 = 1/1000 \qquad 0\cdot005 = 5/1000 = 1/200$$

As can be seen, it is vital to make the decimal point clear and put it in the correct place, with a zero before it to avoid confusion.

The prescription. The use of abbreviations by the doctors is now discouraged and the prescription should be written in full in English, preferably in printed writing.

The drug round

Hospitals determine their own policy on the giving of drugs but two people should be present to check and witness the administration of a drug to a patient.

Procedure. The procedure is as follows:

(1) *Both* nurses, whether qualified or in training, share responsibility for the entire procedure.

(2) No drug of any kind may be given by a nurse unless ordered by a doctor. This includes all the routes by which drugs may be administered.

(3) The prescription sheet must be available and read at the actual time when the drug is checked and given to the patient.

(4) 'Checking' a drug means that both nurses have:
    (*a*) Ensured accuracy in the timing and route of administration.
    (*b*) Measured the exact amount of the correct drug.
    (*c*) Identified the right patient.
    (*d*) Witnessed, i.e. actually watched, the patient swallowing the drug or the injection being given.

(5) Drugs should not be checked first and then set aside to be given later. When a drug is to be given via an intragastric tube the nurse who will give this must take part in the preparation and checking of

the drug. There are a few drugs which may be specifically prescribed by the doctor for self-medication by the individual patient, e.g. glyceryl trinitrate tablets or magnesium trisilicate powder. In this case the patient will be allowed to keep a supply of the drug on his locker.

The expiry date of any drug should always be noted before it is removed from its container together with any special requirements for its storage, e.g. away from the light because of risk of deterioration.

The prescription sheet

Various types of prescription recording systems are in use. They may be in the form of a printed sheet or book. Complete accuracy and adherence to the regulations laid down is essential for safety. It must be remembered that intravenous fluids come into the category of drugs.

Administration of drugs by mouth

Requirements. These are as follows:

Drug trolley and all drugs to be given.
Jug of drinking water.
Medicine measures.
Teaspoons and 5 ml plastic measuring spoons.
Small tray.
Drinking straws if required.
Empty bowl to receive used measures and spoons.
Paper tissues to wipe bottles after use.

Procedure. The procedure is as follows:

(1) The patient is made comfortable before the dose is prepared.

(2) The mixture is poured out; the bottle is held with the label towards the palm of the hand, shaken several times to mix the contents thoroughly and uncapped. Both the bottle and the measure are held at eye level and towards a good light, the prescribed dose is poured out and the cap replaced. The prepared dose is handed to the patient on the small tray and a glass of water offered.

(3) Tablets should not normally be crushed. If the patient cannot swallow tablets or capsules the pharmacist will supply a suitable liquid preparation where possible. Tablets and capsules should not be handled but can be tipped into the bottle cap for counting (for reasons of hygiene and also because of possible allergic effects for

the handler). A separate spoon is used for each patient. Powders may be given from a spoon or folded piece of paper.

(4) Nurses must ensure that the patient swallows the drug.

(5) Bottles are wiped clean and dry after use. Spoons and measures are washed and dried in the kitchen as soon as possible after the drugs have been given.

(6) The drug trolley is locked and then padlocked to the wall again.

Administration of drugs by injection

The patient must be identified and the injection checked by two nurses; this includes the actual insertion of the needle into the patient. When more than one patient is to be given an injection the whole procedure must be carried out separately for each patient concerned. Where more than one drug is prescribed they should never be mixed in the same syringe.

Special precautions with certain drugs. When antibiotics or other substances known to cause hypersensitivity (e.g. chlorpromazine) are being given by injection, clean disposable gloves must always be worn when preparing and giving the injection in order to protect the staff from possible development of dangerous hypersensitivity.

Requirements. These are as follows:

In drawer of trolley:

Assortment of presterilized syringes and needles.
Small gauze swabs.
Ampoule files.
Ampoules of water/sodium chloride 0·9 per cent for injection.
Clean white receivers.
Paper disposal bag.
Disposable gloves.
Chlorhexidine 0·5 per cent and spirit 70 per cent spray.

On lower shelf:

Box for used syringes and needles.

Procedure: The procedure is as follows:

(1) The hands should be socially clean before the equipment is assembled.

(2) The syringe container is opened at the piston end and the needle container at the mount end. The syringe is removed and the needle, still in its container is fixed firmly in place.

(3) The syringe is then charged with the drug. If it has been dispensed in a rubber capped bottle this should first be cleaned with a moistened swab (i.e. from a spray bottle).

(4) Air is expelled from the syringe before withdrawing the needle from the bottle and the needle replaced within protective container. To prevent a vacuum in the bottle, one normally injects in an equivalent volume of air into the bottle. Then the required volume of drug should be drawn into the syringe making sure that no air bubbles are left. The same needle should be used for injecting the drug into the patient. These measures are to prevent the possibility of fine droplets being sprayed into the air, particularly in the case of antibiotic drugs and also to minimize the risk of introducing infection. Care should be taken that the point of the needle is not pressed against the glass of the bottle or ampoule as this may blunt it.

(5) The syringe and attached needle are then placed carefully into the receiver, together with a swab and having replaced the protective cover over the needle it is taken to the patient's bedside and the receiver is placed on the locker. The bed is curtained.

(6) The site for injection is chosen, the patient helped into the most suitable and comfortable position and the injection given after the skin has been cleaned.

(7) The swab is held over the puncture and the needle withdrawn. The swab is then held firmly in position for a moment to seal the puncture and the patient left comfortable.

(8) The nurse washes her hands and the other nurse signs the prescription sheet. The equipment is left clean and ready for use, the receiver is washed or discarded and syringe and needles left *intact* and placed in the sharps box for disposal.

Special points to note about subcutaneous 'hypodermic' injections
(1) Syringes: 1 ml or 2 ml.
(2) Needles: No. 1 (40 mm) serum No. 2 (50 mm), No. 12 (30 mm) or 'serum' needles.
(3) Sites: Outer aspect of arm or thigh.
(4) Method: The tissue is held between thumb and forefinger, and the needle inserted swiftly into the subcutaneous tissue in an upward slanting direction (i.e. at an angle of about thirty degrees to the skin surface).

Special points to note about 'intramuscular' injections
(1) Syringes: 2 ml, 5 ml or 10 ml.

(2) Needles: No. 1 (40 mm) serum No. 2 (50 mm), No. 12 (30 mm) or 'serum' needles. If these injections are to be effective and as painless as possible, they should be given deep into the muscle with a long-bevelled needle at least 40 mm in length. A needle at least 50 mm in length should be used for obese patients, for viscous preparations and for iron preparations.

(3) *Sites:*

(a) The vastus externus muscle, middle third (lateral aspect of thigh). This is not crossed by any important vessel or nerve.

(b) The deltoid muscle for small injections (upper arm, just below point of shoulder).

(c) The gluteus maximus muscle: site must be in the upper and outer quadrant of the buttock to avoid injury to the sciatic nerve.

(4) *Method:*

(a) Ask the patient to relax the muscle.

(b) The skin is made taut by pulling it down firmly with the thumb. (When it returns to its normal position the needle-track will form a zigzag line, preventing leakage of the drug into the subcutaneous tissues.)

(c) The needle is inserted at right angles to the skin with a swift, firm but not stabbing movement, leaving at least 6 mm (0·25 in) of the shaft visible.

(d) The piston is withdrawn slightly to ensure that the needle is not in a blood vessel. If blood appears the needle should be withdrawn slightly and reinserted in a different direction. The hilt of the needle is steadied, the drug injected slowly and the needle withdrawn.

(e) The patient is encouraged to move the muscle as much as possible to aid absorption and prevent pain.

Intravenous administration of drugs

Intravenous injection given normally only by a doctor is used when very quick action is required.

Care of drugs in the home

It is important that when any drugs, including lotions, are kept in the home they should be locked up in a safe place, out of reach of children and given with the same care and accuracy as in hospital.

13

The Surgical Patient

Preoperative Procedure

It is normal to admit the surgical patient at least twenty-four hours before his operation is to be performed. This allows time for him to learn a little about ward routine and to meet the people who will be looking after him so that after his operation he returns to familiar surroundings. During this time the medical staff can carry out a thorough examination of the patient and the anaesthetist too is given the opportunity to check on the patient's condition.

Written consent is needed whether the operation is to be performed under general or local anaesthesia and though the doctor is responsible the nurse must check that the consent form has been signed. For patients under sixteen years, consent of parent or guardian must be obtained. If the patient is mentally or physically incapable of signing for himself it is usual for a close relative to do so.

Preparation of the patient

Diet and drugs. Special diet or *regimen* of drugs may have been ordered and early admission may be necessary to ensure that the regimen is followed. It is important that the stomach is empty before general anaesthesia and this means that the patient is not allowed food or drink six hours before operation; the anaesthetist may give specific instructions. Special bowel preparation may be ordered according to: the operation, the time available, the surgeon's wishes and the age and general condition of the patient.

The skin. The operation site must be cleaned very thoroughly and this includes shaving all hair in the area. The skin must not be nicked or cut and care must be taken to leave on the body any marks put there by the surgeon. A bactericidal solution may be used instead of soap but talcum powder must not be applied.

Immediate preparation

The patient passes urine and then has a bath or shower (or blanket bath), special attention being paid to the nails, the umbilicus, skin folds and the operation area. Cosmetics are removed and prostheses such as spectacles or contact lenses, artificial eyes and false teeth, jewellery, hairclips and wigs etc. are put into the patient's locker. Internal tampons and sanitary belts are removed and replaced with a clean sanitary towel and bandage. While the patient is bathing the operation bed is prepared. A carrier for dirty bed linen is taken to the bedside with the following clean articles:

(1) Theatre gown.
(2) Long cotton socks.
(3) Flannelette blanket.
(4) Cotton blanket.
(5) Drawsheet.
(6) Pillowcases.
(7) Theatre canvas.

Every hospital has its own rules to suit its circumstances and though this is a general minimal list, a cotton or paper cap, head blanket and antistatic mackintosh may also be needed.

The patient is usually taken to the theatre suite on a trolley though if he is very ill or unable to move easily he may be taken to the theatre suite in his bed.

Premedication. Two nurses give the premedication checking drug and dose as for any other medication. In addition they ensure that:

(1) The urine has been tested and recorded.
(2) The notes and X-rays are together.
(3) The consent form has been signed.
(4) The wrist bracelet details are correct.
(5) The premedication form has been checked and signed by both nurses.
(6) Dental reconstructions are noted on the form.
(7) Any known reactions are noted, e.g. to iodine or Elastoplast.

The patient is reassured as necessary and observed for any reactions to the premedication; for this purpose curtains may be drawn on either side of his bed but not at the foot.

Taking the patient to theatre. The theatre porter brings the trolley into the ward and shows the theatre slip, which bears the patient's name, to the sister or nurse in charge. A ward nurse accompanies the patient (walking near his head) and on arrival at the anaesthetic room checks with the theatre staff that the right patient has been brought. The nurse stays until her patient is unconscious and even then leaves only when the theatre sister has given permission for her to do so. Some operations are performed under local or spinal anaesthesia and as the patient may be conscious the nurse will be asked to stay with him in the theatre.

Postoperative Care

The nurse accompanying the patient from the recovery room or theatre should take a set of postanaesthetic instruments, namely:

(1) Mouth gag.
(2) Tongue forceps.
(3) Sponge-holding forceps.
(4) Tongue depressor.
(5) Wooden wedge.
(6) Receiver for swabs.

Before she leaves the recovery room with her patient she satisfies herself that the patient's colour, respiration and pulse are satisfactory. She also checks the operation site dressing. She is told what operation has been carried out and is given details of the anaesthetic, drainage tubes and instructions given by the anaesthetist or surgeon. She also collects the patient's notes and prescription sheets.

On the way back to the ward the nurse is responsible for the patient's airway and general safety on the trolley. She keeps him covered, looks after any apparatus such as an intravenous infusion and watches the patient's colour and respiration. As soon as he has returned to the ward the patient is lifted into his bed and if his condition allows, is turned to one side so that the theatre canvas, mackintosh and draw-sheet can be rolled together and removed from the bed to go back to the theatre. The patient is settled into a position suitable to his operation, age and condition. This may be semi-prone or sitting up with the backrest raised. A bed cradle will take the weight of the bed-clothes. The nurse now reports the patient's arrival to the ward sister and gives the details she received when she fetched the patient. While the patient is unconscious a nurse stays with him to: —

(1) Maintain the airway.
(2) Protect the restless patient from injury.

(3) Observe pulse, respiration, colour and operation site and record.

(4) Manage equipment.

Good lighting is required so that the nurse can see at once even slight changes in his appearance.

Postoperative complications

Respiration. Airway obstruction may be caused by vomit or blood from the throat entering the larynx when the patient inhales, or by the tongue falling back. Breathing may fail because of the depressing effect of the anaesthetic and narcotic drugs on the respiratory centre in the brain. Should either occur, immediate action is needed.

Haemorrhage. Regular examination of the dressing is essential. If internal haemorrhage occurs, the first signs are of increasing pallor and a rising pulse rate. The patient's pulse should be taken at regular intervals after the operation to ensure early detection of this.

Shock is a very severe condition which cannot always be readily compensated. It arises from the fact that there is less blood in circulation than could fill all the blood vessels if they were to remain open; normally the autonomic nervous system controls the veins and arteries very precisely and the brain, heart and kidneys continue to receive their required amount of blood but those organs not essential to immediate survival, namely the muscles, stomach, intestines and skin, receive a very reduced volume. If for any reason this corrective mechanism fails, less blood gets to the heart, so that its output is reduced, blood pressure falls and the pulse rate increases. The patient may feel his heart pounding away, he becomes frightened and the situation becomes even worse.

The causes of shock may be physical or mental and the patient is given drugs to allay preoperative anxiety and is handled and talked to kindly and gently. The surgeon operates gently and may use only local anaesthesia during the operation. Haemorrhage is a cause of shock and blood lost is replaced as soon as possible.

By a careless word or showing your alarm you can rapidly induce shock in your patient. For sound medical reasons you must remain calm in a postoperative emergency; calm, competent and quick.

Discomfort. There are several conditions which initially cause discomfort though not immediate danger. Postanaesthetic vomiting may prove dangerous if it persists and a dilated stomach may be associated with it; a naso-oesophageal tube should prevent either occurring. Urine retention may be treated by warming the lower abdomen, giving a hot drink and allowing men patients to stand out of bed. Catheterization is not to be thought of as the normal initial treatment. Pain is treated with drugs which may be continued for some time if movement is desirable but which would otherwise prove impossible to the patient.

14

Emergencies in the Ward

Every hospital has an emergency procedure which will be explained to all hospital staff. It may involve the use of wireless 'bleepers', alarm bells, lights or the telephone.

There are three situations when only immediate action by the nurse or indeed anyone else at hand can save a patient's life; 'immediate' meaning within four minutes. If the supply of oxygen to the brain ceases and is not renewed within four minutes the brain will be so severely damaged that it can never be entirely efficient again. There may be loss of use of a limb, of speech or of eyesight even if the patient seems to recover. Two things are vital—speed and action. You are on your own, for that moment at least.

An emergency arises when:

(1) The patient stops breathing.
(2) The patient's heart stops.
(3) Severe bleeding is seen.

Respiratory Failure

This may be caused by:

(1) Obstruction of the respiratory passages or lungs.
(2) Collapse of the lungs.
(3) Paralysis of the respiratory muscles.
(4) Paralysis of the nerve centre controlling the respiratory muscles.

Look at the patient's chest to see if it is moving. If it is not, put your ear close to his nose and mouth and listen. If you cannot hear anything clear his airway and start mouth-to-mouth breathing. Fresh air contains twenty-one per cent oxygen, whilst expired air contains eighteen per cent. Thus the air you breathe into your patient still has plenty of oxygen.

To clear the patient's airway:

(1) Take out his dentures.

(2) Wrap a handkerchief round your finger, turn his head to one side, and run your finger round inside his mouth to remove vomit, blood, water or any other obstruction.

(3) Bend his head back as far as it will go. At the same time bring his lower jaw up until his teeth are firmly closed and hold it there. This prevents the unconscious patient's tongue falling back and blocking his throat.

Mouth-to-mouth breathing. Lay the patient on his back. Bend his head fully back and draw his lower jaw upwards. Close his nostrils with your other hand. Take a deep breath and making an airtight seal with your mouth over the patient's mouth, blow into him. Take your mouth away and look sideways to see that his chest is falling as the air escapes from his lungs. Repeat this process about twelve times a minute. If the patient is a child fit your mouth over both his mouth and his nose and be very gentle as you breathe into him, otherwise you may damage his lungs. Go on with mouth-to-mouth breathing until the patient is breathing himself or until a doctor tells you to stop.

Cardiac Arrest

Closed-chest cardiac massage is a means of restarting a heart which has stopped. In the unconscious patient whose breathing has stopped massage should be started if:

(1) There is no visible improvement after six inflations.

(2) No pulse can be felt.

(3) The pupils are widely dilated.

(4) Death appears imminent.

The principle is to squeeze the heart between the backbone and the lower part of the sternum so that blood is expelled into the circulation; relaxing the pressure allows the heart to fill again. The patient must be on his back on a hard surface; cardiac massage on a soft bed is totally ineffectual. If a board is ready at hand, place it beneath the patient, otherwise heave him onto the floor or any hard surface.

(1) Kneel beside the patient. You must be able to lean over him so that your shoulders with your arms straight are above the middle of the chest.

(2) Feel for the breast bone, the sternum, find its mid-point and place the heel of one hand between this point and the lower end of the sternum.

(3) Place the second hand over the first.

(4) Lean forward so that with straight arms your shoulders are directly above the patient's chest.

(5) Press down firmly and quickly so as to depress the breast bone 3–4 cm (1–2 in).

(6) Quickly release the pressure.

(7) Repeat at one second intervals; say to yourself 'one thousand', press–release, 'two thousand', press–release and so on.

Haemorrhage

Haemorrhage is the loss of blood from any part of the body. It may be external and easily seen or internal. In both events prompt action is necessary or your patient may die in a very few minutes.

External bleeding

Treatment is simple. Apply pressure to the place from which blood is flowing and use any form of cloth to help staunch the flow. You are dealing with a lifesaving procedure which does not allow you time to find, unpack and apply a sterile dressing. Do not apply a tourniquet, do not look for pressure points but raise the part which is bleeding and hold your temporary dressing firmly in place.

Internal bleeding

This always requires a doctor's attention. The nurse's primary role is to recognize that internal bleeding is occurring and to reassure the patient who will become frightened when he becomes aware of what is happening.

Haemoptysis. Bright red and frothy blood is coughed up. This indicates that the blood is from the lungs and arises from injury or a lung disease such as tuberculosis or carcinoma.

Haematemesis. Blood is vomited. Blood that has been in the stomach for some time and has been partially digested by gastric juices is dark and contains particles.

15

Bandages, Splints and Slings

Bandages

Bandages may be applied for a number of reasons, and the kind of bandage used will usually depend on the purpose of its application. They may include triangular bandages, crêpe (elastic) bandages, adhesive elastic bandages, adhesive plasters and Tubegauz.

The purpose of a bandage may be to:

(1) Keep dressings in place.
(2) Give steady support to a part.
(3) Stop bleeding by applying pressure.
(4) Prevent movement.
(5) Speed venous return.

Rules for applying roller bandages:

(1) Place the limb in the position it will occupy when bandaged.

(2) Put absorbent wool or some soft material between any surfaces that would otherwise be in contact and over bony areas.

(3) Secure the beginning of the bandage by two straight turns round the limb.

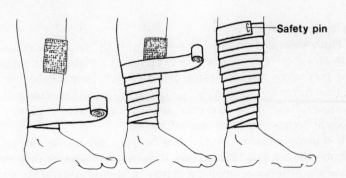

Fig. 4. Application of a roller bandage to the leg.

(4) Bandage from below upwards, and from within outwards. Each turn should overlap two-thirds of the preceding one.

(5) Do not apply a bandage to a limb so tightly that the limb beyond becomes painful, numb, swollen, white or blue.

(6) Do not bandage so loosely as to serve no purpose; in addition a loose bandage slips and is uncomfortable.

(7) Ensure that the bandage is dry; a damp one will shrink and become tight.

Triangular bandages

These may be used for slings, to apply splints, or to hold dressings in place but their use, except for slings, is mainly confined to first aid.

Crêpe (elastic) bandages

These are cotton bandages which have elastic properties but contain no rubber elastic; their elasticity is due to the way they were woven. Crêpe bandages fit closely and comfortably to all the different parts of the body and are used not only to hold dressings in place but also to give support, e.g. in sprains. They can be washed frequently and are thus economical.

Adhesive elastic bandages

These bandages, e.g. Elastoplast, are made of cotton material, woven to have elastic properties like crêpe bandages but with an adhesive zinc substance applied to them. They are often used for the support of varicose ulcers and are applied directly to the skin in an upward spiral direction.

Adhesive plasters

These consist of plastic cotton material with one side impregnated with an adhesive substance. There are many varieties on the market and they often take the place of bandages which can be hot and bulky. Adhesive plaster is particularly useful to cover finger dressings. Sellotape is sometimes used as an alternative, though this tends to become hard and uncomfortable.

Removing adhesive plasters can be very painful for the patient because the hairs on the skin may be torn out. To lessen this, always shave the skin before applying plaster in any quantity. Take a swab dipped in ether (which is used as a solvent), raise a small corner of the plaster, press the swab hard against the uncovered skin and pull the plaster back several centimetres. Move the swab close up against the plaster again and rip back another section. It will be found that the cold of the ether distracts the patient's attention for a moment, while pressing hard on the skin keeps it tight whilst ripping the plaster rather than gently pulling it off will make it unlikely that the patient will feel very much at all.

Tubegauz

This is a form of bandaging now used in many hospitals and doctors' surgeries. A nurse, with a little practice, should soon be able to use it quickly and efficiently. Tubegauz is a machine knitted cotton bandage prepared in the form of a tube which is applied by means of a series of metal applicators. There are various sizes of both bandage and applicator to fit all parts of the body. These applicators hold lengths of tubular bandage which may be cut off to the size required after being passed several times over the area to be covered.

Splints

Splints may be straight or moulded to the shape of the injured part. Those most commonly used now are light, pliable splints made of Perspex or other plastic material, held in place by bandages. They may also be moulded in plaster of Paris or, in an emergency, any stiff object such as a rolled newspaper or umbrella may be used.

Plaster bandages

These can be bought already prepared and impregnated with plaster of Paris. They are immersed in cool water and applied while still wet. When dry a hard shell is formed and in this way fractured limbs, etc. can be immobilized to give them complete rest.

Care of a patient in a plaster of Paris bandage

If a patient has a fracture which is treated by the application of a plaster and has to stay in bed at least for a while the bedclothes and pillows should be protected with polythene or mackintosh sheets. Air should be allowed to circulate freely round the plaster to help it to dry. This can be achieved by putting a bedcradle over the plaster and the bedclothes over it. Direct heat should not be applied as quick drying of the plaster could cause it to crack.

The plaster should be examined regularly and the limb watched to see that toes or fingers do not look blue, feel cold or numb and that pressure lesions do not occur.

Fracture boards should always be put into a bed for the patient to keep the bed firm and give support to the limb.

Preparation for the application of plaster of Paris:

Requirements. These are as follows:
For the surgeon:
Mackintosh apron.
Gown.
Rubber gloves.
Cotton leggings or gum boots.

Mackintoshes to protect the bed and the floor.
Shaving equipment.
Powder for the limb
Stockinette.
Sheet wadding or thick padding of wool if there is likely to be much swelling.
Large bowl of tepid water for soaking the bandages (unless the bowl is of plastic it should be thinly coated inside with petroleum jelly to prevent the plaster from sticking to it).
Plaster of Paris bandages.

Tray with:
Tape measure.
Blue pencil.
Scissors.
Plaster shears, knives and scissors if an old plaster needs removing.

Points to be remembered in the application of plaster.
(1) Shave the limb, powder it and cover with stockinette or wool.
(2) Hold the limb steady throughout the application and be careful not to press on the wet plaster and use the flat of the hand, not the fingers.
(3) Trim and turn up the bandages over the edges, polish and leave smooth.
(4) After the plaster is dry, watch for any blueness of the extremities and report any complaint of coldness, numbness or pain. These symptoms are indication of interference with the circulation.

It should be remembered that pressure deadens sensation and that the skin may be pressed upon and that bedsores may develop.

A nurse must never cut or interfere with plaster. If a patient complains of the above symptoms a doctor must be informed.

No patient should be sent home with a new plaster on without being told when to report for examination and he must be told to return at once if he is worried or unduly uncomfortable, if his toes or fingers swell or look blue, feel cold or hurt. A printed form of instructions should be given to the patient or his nearest relative before he leaves the hospital.

Simple Slings

It is often necessary to support the injured arm or hand of a patient who is fully ambulant and well. A strained muscle will be rested and the throbbing sensation in a badly cut finger eased if the hand is raised and the elbow supported.

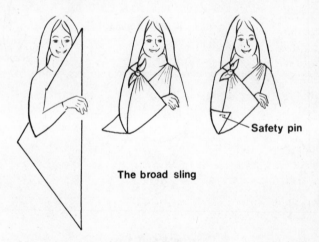

Safety pin

The broad sling

Fig. 5. Triangular bandage used as a sling to support the arm; note the position of the knot.

The broad sling, Fig. 5, leaves the hand free but the weight of the arm is taken over the back of the neck which may become tired after several hours.

The St. John's sling, Fig. 6, supports the hand and prevents it being used. It is particularly useful in patients who want to ignore their injuries. Its additional advantage lies in the fact that its position across the back provides a very restful support.

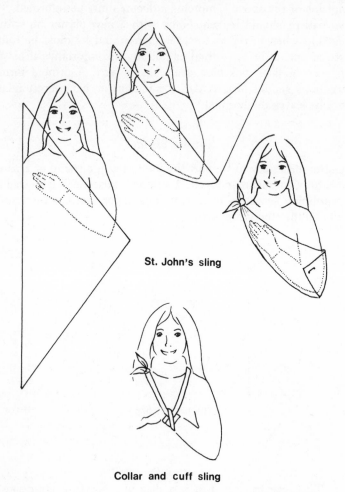

St. John's sling

Collar and cuff sling

Fig. 6. Triangular bandage supporting hand and arm and below, a simple sling which can be put on by the patient.

The collar and cuff sling can be made from a bandage or necktie; it can be put on by the patient himself, removed when necessary and replaced.

16

Infection

Infection results from the presence in or on the body of pathogenic micro-organisms which give rise to clinical symptoms of disease. Many micro-organisms are found in the body, particularly on the skin and in the gut, which are harmless at these sites; these are called commensals. Commensals can become pathogenic when they are transmitted to an abnormal site such as a wound or the bladder.

The following are the main types of micro-organism causing disease:

Bacteria. These are divided into aerobes, which require oxygen to survive, and anaerobes, which only flourish without oxygen. Bacteria can be further classified according to the different shapes which can be identified under the microscope:

Bacilli: Rod-shaped organisms examples of which are tetanus and tuberculosis.

Cocci: Round organisms. Examples of these are *Streptococcus* and *Staphylococcus.*

Spirilla: Spiral organisms, for example the spirochaete of syphilis.

Certain groups of bacterial micro-organisms, such as those responsible for anthrax, tetanus and gas gangrene, are capable of producing spores which can survive for long periods without food or moisture and can resist wide changes in temperature. They will lie dormant until conditions become suitable for their growth.

Viruses. These are micro-organisms so small that only the larger ones can be seen through the ordinary microscope. The smaller ones may be detected by an electron microscope. Viruses are responsible for many diseases among which are poliomyelitis, measles and influenza as well as the common cold.

Fungi. These forms of vegetable life may cause infections such as ringworm and athletes' foot.

Methods of Treating Disease Caused by Micro-organisms

Bacterial infections. The modern method of treating bacterial disease is by the use of antibiotics, themselves produced by other bacteria or moulds. There are many antibiotics in use in medicine today and the number is constantly increasing. In order to be sure that the correct antibiotic is being used to treat a particular disease, it is necessary to take a swab from the infected site and send it correctly labelled and with the accompanying form, to the pathological laboratory so that it may be incubated and identified and its sensitivity to a particular antibiotic demonstrated. As this process may take up to forty-eight hours, after the swab has been taken the doctor will probably order a broad-spectrum antibiotic such as ampicillin to be administered to the patient, if the infection is severe, whilst he is awaiting the results of the tests.

A broad-spectrum antibiotic is one which acts against a wide range of bacteria. However, because it is not selective it affects beneficial as well as pathogenic bacteria and its use is discontinued as soon as the pathogen is identified. The specific antibiotic can then be prescribed.

Viral infections. The majority of viruses do not respond to treatment with antibiotics. For instance it is useless to attempt to treat influenza with penicillin or any other antibiotic. When dealing with patients suffering from viral infections, good nursing is the most important factor. The diseases are usually self-limiting so that spontaneous recovery will commonly occur in the absence of a further infection such as bronchitis or pneumonia.

Fungal infections. It is possible to treat fungal infections by specific antifungal agents such as nystatin and griseofulvin. All antifungal agents, except in fact griseofulvin, are applied locally to the site involved.

Inflammation

Inflammation is the response of the body to trauma and is evidence that the body is reacting to bacterial or viral invasion or to physical change.

The cardinal signs of inflammation are redness, heat, swelling, pain and loss of function. Some infections, such as a boil or stye may be localized, but generalized infections, for instance, pneumonia, will also produce a raised body temperature with muscle pains, alternate feelings of hotness and intense shivering (rigor) and general malaise.

The mechanism by which the body defends itself against infection is by mobilization of white blood corpuscles to the affected site. These white blood corpuscles are called phagocytes and are capable of ingesting the invading bacteria. The resulting products may be eliminated from the body either through the lymphatic system or, in certain more superficial infections such as boils, by the discharge of pus.

Antibodies

The body has the ability to recognize the entry of foreign proteins such as bacteria or viruses, which are known as antigens, and will respond by producing an antibody which will destroy the activity of the antigen. The self-limiting diseases referred to earlier such as measles and influenza are examples of this mechanism. Furthermore, in some diseases, once the antibody has been produced it will confer lasting immunity against the disease should it be encountered on future occasions. However this does not hold true for all disease processes and in some cases, although the body may produce antibodies to the infecting organism, it may not in itself be capable of bringing the infection under control. In such a case, chemotherapy must be employed, as described in the section on bacterial infections. Moreover in these cases, the antibodies produced may not confer lasting immunity and the patient may suffer repeated attacks of the disease.

Vaccination and Immunization

As already described immunity is acquired through the production of antibodies in response to an infection. Immunization may also be stimulated by the injection of vaccines prepared from dead or attenuated organisms. Whilst a vaccine does not induce the disease, the presence of these dead organisms stimulates the production of antibodies to it. In this way immunity is conferred before a person comes into contact with the disease and he is thus protected.

The policy in the United Kingdom of vaccination from infancy has resulted in the virtual elimination of certain diseases such as smallpox, diphtheria and poliomyelitis and has greatly reduced the incidence of whooping cough, measles, tetanus and tuberculosis. Girls of twelve to thirteen years of age are now immunized against rubella to eliminate any risk to the fetus in future pregnancies and measles vaccine is given to babies of twelve to fourteen months.

Since international travel is now so common, travellers to or from certain countries where these diseases occur are required to produce evidence of vaccination against smallpox, cholera and yellow fever and in some cases it is desirable that the individual should be protected against typhoid fever and exceptionally rabies, typhus and plague. Thus it will be seen that modern methods of immunization by vaccination have gone a long way to conquer traditional life-threatening diseases such as smallpox and diphtheria.

Spread of Infection

Micro-organisms can enter the body in various ways and once a person has been invaded by infection there is a risk that it may be passed to others in the following ways:

(1) By inhalation of droplets through the mouth and nose which spread to the respiratory tract. By this method influenza, the common cold and tuberculosis may be contracted.

(2) By ingestion of pathogenic micro-organisms which will be carried into the alimentary tract, for example gastroenteritis, dysentery and poliomyelitis.

Contaminated water may be a source of infections such as typhoid fever, dysentery and cholera although with the greatly improved sanitation of modern times in western Europe outbreaks of these diseases are most unlikely to occur. Milk may be responsible for outbreaks of any of these diseases and may carry living tubercle bacilli, though here again the tuberculin testing of cattle and pasteurization of milk in this country has eliminated this method of spread of infection.

(3) By inoculation through the skin and mucous membrane to the tissue beneath. Many infections may enter the body in this way and it is important for the nurse to remember that if she has, say, an infected finger or a boil she is capable of causing a severe infection in the wound of a patient.

Food may become contaminated by certain organisms occasionally resulting in food poisoning, the most common organisms being the *Salmonella* group. Foods most frequently affected are meat pies, sausages and meat pastes but any food that has been handled frequently, or that has been inadequately cooked for a second time may be responsible for infection. It is most important that all food handlers should observe strict hygiene particularly, for example, those working in food manufacturing concerns or canteens. They should be free from infection such as that resulting from carious teeth or infected ears. Nurses should always be careful to wash their hands before handling food.

Infection may be carried by flies and other insects such as fleas, bugs and lice. The 'Black Death', or plague, in medieval England was carried by fleas harboured by the brown rat that was brought to the country by ship. Plague is still endemic in parts of India and East Africa. Occasionally infection may be spread by a carrier, that is, a person harbouring an infection without any clinical symptoms or who has recovered from an attack without the elimination of the causative organism. The classic examples of this are streptococci found in the nose and throat of apparently healthy people (known as carriers) and, in the past, typhoid fever organisms passed in the stool.

Types of outbreaks of infectious diseases

Outbreaks of infectious diseases may be classified according to type as follows:

(1) Sporadic, where a limited number of widely separated people are affected.

(2) Epidemic, where a large number of cases occur in one area for a limited time.

(3) Endemic, where a disease occurs constantly in one area over a long period.

Cross-infection

This term refers to the passing of an infection from one person to another in a specific environment such as a hospital ward where patients are particularly susceptible to infection by micro-organisms that they may not have encountered previously and to which they have no immunity. Many hospitals now have Control of Infection Officers, who may be specially chosen nurses, whose job it is to see that the conditions that may favour the spread of infection are reduced to the minimum.

There are many factors to be considered in the prevention of cross-infection in hospital and these include clean, well-ventilated wards with the beds adequately spaced. In 1968 the Department of Health and Social Security recommended that bed centres should be at least 8 ft (2·5 m approx.) apart with a minimum distance of 6·5 ft (2 m approx.) between bed ends opposite to each other. Most new hospitals are designed to provide smaller wards (four to eight beds) with many more single rooms.

Adequate washing facilities should be provided for patients and staff and the simple rules of hygiene scrupulously observed. The patient should be encouraged to wash his hands after using a urinal, bedpan, commode or W.C. (the nurse should bring a bowl of water if he is confined to bed). Nurses should always remember to wash their hands after handling a bedpan or urinal and before and after carrying out dressings or giving injections. Other measures include the proper cleaning of wards; vacuum cleaners should be used to pick up dust from floors, surfaces should be easy to clean with no awkward corners in which dust can collect and dusting should be carried out using a damp cloth. On beds cotton blankets are preferable to woollen ones as they can be laundered more adequately and because the action of bed-making causes dust that may contain millions of micro-organisms to fly into the air, at least one hour should elapse before dressings are carried out. Dirty dressings are placed in the bags provided and burnt in the incinerator and dirty linen is put into bags for collection by the laundry porter. Infected linen should be treated separately and should be placed in bags that are clearly labelled. Paper towels should be provided in ward kitchens and beside washbasins, and paper handkerchiefs should be used and then discarded. A nurse who has a minor infection such as a cold, sore throat, septic finger or any other infection should report it at once.

Prevention of the spread of infection

All cases of infectious diseases must be reported to the Area Specialist in Environmental Health. Steps will then be taken to contain the infection by:

(1) Tracing the source of infection and removing it. If it is caused, say, by contaminated food this may be a comparatively simple matter.

(2) Isolating the patient with the disease and giving the appropriate treatment.

(3) Tracing the contacts of the infected patient, giving prophylactic treatment where indicated and if necessary isolating contacts for as long as there is any danger of infection being passed on.

The complete list of diseases that are compulsorily notifiable in the United Kingdom is:

Acute meningitis	Plague
Anthrax	Acute poliomyelitis
Cholera	Undulant fever
Diphtheria	Scarlet fever
Dysentery (amoebic or bacillary)	Smallpox
Acute encephalitis	Tetanus
Food poisoning	Tuberculosis
Infective jaundice	Typhoid and paratyphoid
Leptospirosis	fever
Leprosy	Typhus
Malaria	Whooping cough
Measles	Yellow fever
Ophthalmia neonatorum	

A number of these diseases are unlikely to be encountered in this country but may be introduced by travellers from abroad, particularly from Africa and Asia: examples are malaria and cholera; others such as smallpox and diphtheria have been controlled in Britain by immunization.

In many cases patients with simple infectious conditions may be nursed at home but should be isolated as far as possible from other vulnerable members of the family. With rubella, which in itself is a mild infection, it may be thought desirable to expose young girls in the family to the infection because if the disease is contracted before childbearing age danger in any future pregnancy may be avoided.

Some patients with acute infectious diseases are best nursed in a special hospital for infectious conditions. However, if the patient is admitted to a general ward strict precautions must be taken by barrier nursing to prevent the spread of infection to other patients.

Barrier nursing

The principles of barrier nursing are directed towards the isolation of the patient from others and the prevention of transfer of the infection outside the barrier. Such nursing is best carried out in a single room or cubicle, but where this is not possible a bed may be screened and all articles used in connection with the patient kept within the screens. The infectious patient is best nursed in a single room, and the techniques employed can be adapted to the 'barrier' within the ward.

(1) The number of nursing staff should be reduced to a minimum and the number of visitors restricted. Gowns should be worn by all who enter the room and masks too if the infection is airborne. Gowns should be of the disposable type where possible, but if not disposable should be taken off carefully, avoiding touching the contaminated outside of the gown and left in the room. Masks should be disposed of after each wearing and should never be worn for more than twenty minutes without a change as they become saturated with expired air.

(2) All equipment used in the care of the patient should be kept inside the room with the exception of charts which should be kept outside.

(3) Cleaning of the room should be carried out under nursing supervision. In addition to cleaning the floor with a vacuum cleaner kept just for this room and containing an inner lining which can be disposed of, all surfaces should be wiped with a disinfectant solution using disposable cloths such as a J cloth, or a paper towel.

(4) There should be facilities for washing within the room and doctors, nurses and visitors should wash their hands on entering and before leaving the room.

(5) When serving meals to the patient, disposable plates, cups and utensils should be used where practicable or the patient should have his own china and cutlery which is washed in the room and kept there. All food left over should be put in the special bin with the other articles for incineration.

(6) Where the infection may be passed through the patient's excreta or sputum, disposable containers should be used and the excreta incinerated. Where such facilities do not exist, excreta must be thoroughly disinfected for a recorded time before being disposed of.

(7) Bed linen should be placed in a special container and autoclaved before being sent to the laundry.

(8) Terminal cleaning of the room should be thorough and all articles used during the patient's stay disinfected. Linen, blankets and pillows should be autoclaved and if necessary the room should be fumigated.

Reverse barrier nursing

In the case of patients who have no natural defence to combat micro-organisms 'reverse barrier nursing' may be employed. This type of patient includes those who have undergone transplant surgery and those receiving immunosuppressive therapy. The underlying principle is to protect the patient from infection coming from outside.

The techniques of reverse barrier nursing include filtering the air coming into the room from outside the building, thorough cleaning of the room before it is occupied by the patient and the provision of new or sterilized equipment. Anyone entering the room must wear mask and gown and must observe scrupulous personal hygiene. The number of people allowed into the room should be kept to a minimum.

Methods of killing micro-organisms

In the early days of surgery no attention was paid to what is now called surgical cleanliness because the cause of sepsis was not understood. Surgeons commonly operated in frock coats and would wipe their instruments clean on the tails of the coat before proceeding to the next case. Since the discovery of the existence of micro-organisms causing infection methods have been found to prevent their entry into wounds. This is known as *asepsis* (absence of sepsis).

The cleaning and sterilization of articles in common use

After use, articles that have been in contact with blood, pus and other excreta from the body, which all contain protein, should first be rinsed well in cold water because protein coagulates in contact with hot water.

Until comparatively recent times the most common method of sterilizing certain articles such as glass and metal syringes (with the glass wrapped in gauze or old linen to prevent breakage), stainless steel, enamel and rubber equipment, including rubber gloves, was to boil them in a sterilizer in the ward. The articles to be treated should be immersed completely in cold water, care being taken to expel all air, brought to the boil and boiled for five minutes. They should then be removed from the sterilizer using Cheatle forceps that are kept beside the sterilizer in an antiseptic solution. This is not a very satisfactory method as although it will kill most micro-organisms, those that are spore-forming, for example the tetanus bacillus, are resistant. However in hospitals and clinics where more

Bas-il-us

sophisticated methods are not available it may still be necessary to use a sterilizer.

Other methods of sterilization include:

Irradiation by gamma rays. This method is widely used to sterilize the disposable dressings and instruments which are in wide use today.

Autoclaving. The autoclave will produce steam under pressure which will produce temperatures up to 134°C (273°F). Articles to be sterilized by this method should be wrapped loosely in packs which will allow the steam to penetrate.

Dry Heat. A hot air oven is used where articles cannot be penetrated by steam. This is suitable for glass, powder and oils.

Chemical agents which may be divided into:

(1) *Detergents* for cleaning purposes, for example hexachlorophene, which can be used for washing the hands in operating theatres and other clinical situations. For this purpose it is combined with a suitable soap.

(2) *Antiseptics* which inhibit the growth of micro-organisms but do not kill them (bacteriostats). An example of an antiseptic is Eusol, a chlorinated lime and boric acid compound which can be used for dressing wounds.

(3) *Disinfectants* which will kill micro-organisms (bactericides), for example Sudol, an emulsified solution of a cresol compound suitable for floors, surfaces and the soaking of infected linen. This has largely replaced the use of Lysol which is an irritant and must be used with great care.

Central sterile supply department. From early in the 1960s the trend has been towards the establishment in hospitals of Central Sterile Supply Departments (CSSD). These departments are designed and staffed specifically to cope with the cleaning, packaging and re-sterilization of instruments and equipment for the wards, operating theatres and departments of hospitals and have almost completely taken over this function from the wards. Thus a high and uniform standard of sterility is maintained and the nursing staff are freed to give more attention to their patients.

Nursing a Patient with a Fever

When a patient has a fever the heat regulating centre in the brain is affected. Pyrexia ensues producing temperatures from 37° to 39·4°C

(99–103°F). There may be many causes but infection of some kind is the commonest. The patient feels generally unwell, hot, yet cold and shivery, and usually has a headache. He should be put to rest in bed in a well-ventilated room without draughts and, if his headache is bad, he may like to have the curtains drawn to keep out bright light.

The patient may perspire profusely as his temperature falls and his sheets and clothing become a source of great discomfort when they are soaked in perspiration. So it is essential to have clean sheets and a change of night attire available. In some cases flannelette sheets can be used instead of cotton ones as they absorb moisture much better. The mattress may be protected with polythene or rubber sheeting. A drawsheet adds to the patient's comfort, as it can be pulled through and a cool part of the sheet is then available for the patient to lie on.

He should have a blanket bath every day with particular care given to his axillae and groins and to any areas subject to pressure. Talcum powder helps the patient to feel cool and fresh. The hair should be well brushed and, if long, kept off the face, if the patient is a woman it can be tied back with ribbon. The nurse should remember that when the patient perspires the hair becomes moist as well as the skin.

Fluid loss as a result of perspiration makes the patient feel thirsty and his mouth becomes dry. It is important to encourage him to drink as much as possible. It does not matter what he drinks so long as enough is taken. Drinks may be made as attractive as possible, e.g. orange juice may have ice added to it. Drinking straws or feeders may be useful as they allow the patient to drink in a more relaxed and comfortable position.

Particular care must be given to the patient's mouth, because if it is allowed to become dry the tongue and lips become cracked and this may cause sores to develop round the mouth and lead to local infection. The patient's breath may smell and this is called halitosis.

To begin with the patient will only be able to tolerate a liquid diet but as his condition improves he should be able to eat a light diet which can be easily digested. This would include dishes made of milk, eggs lightly boiled, egg custard, bread and butter etc.

Accurate records of the patient's condition must be kept, and his temperature, pulse and respiration recorded four-hourly. Any change should be reported and entered in the record book. If urinary output is poor this must be reported and the volume charted.

The patient may be prescribed antibiotics or antipyretics (to lower the temperature), e.g. Aspirin. These must be given as ordered.

Remember that the patient may be confused and anxious and will need constant supervision and reassurance.

If the patient is suffering from a specific infectious disease, e.g. measles, or chicken-pox, the same nursing principles will apply, but in addition precautions must be taken to prevent the spread of infection.

17

Nursing Care of the Young

In the course of her work a nurse looks after people of all ages, children, adolescents, adults and elderly. Each of these groups have their own needs and problems.

Looking After Babies

The normal infant

The normal infant weighs just over 3 kg (7 lb approx.) at birth. As a rule the baby loses a few ounces (100 to 200 g) of its birth-weight during the first three days but soon regains it. He should gain about 6 oz (200 g) a week in the first three months, after which he progresses at a slightly slower rate. The normal weight for a child of one year is about 9·5 kg (21 lb) and for a child of six years about 20·4 kg (45 lb).

About the end of the fourth month the baby will be able to distinguish objects with his eyes. He will be disturbed by loud or sudden noises, although more gentle sounds are only gradually appreciated.

A baby should begin to lift up his head by the fourth month; at six months he should sit comfortably without support. At ten months he should be able to stand with support and at twelve months he should begin to talk. From twelve to eighteen months he should begin to walk.

Sleep is very important in mental and physical development. The baby must be placed comfortably in his cot, with light and warm covering but no pillow. There should be plenty of cool (16°C, 55°F) fresh air without draughts. An infant should sleep whenever he is not being fed, bathed or having exercise. Until he is four years old a child needs a sleep during the day, as well as at night. If a child is left in the open air to sleep, care must be taken to protect him from the sun as his skin is delicate and burns easily.

The child should have all his first teeth by the age of two and a half. Eruption of the second teeth starts at about six years of age, and by the twelfth year all but wisdom teeth are present.

Exercise. The older baby needs exercise so that his muscles and limbs may develop properly. He should be put on a blanket in the playpen or other safe place and allowed to kick freely for about half an hour at least twice a day, before a feed is due.

Clothing should be suitable for the season and should be light in weight, warm and absorbent. Overclothing causes rashes, sweating and dehydration. Care must be taken to shield a baby's head and ears from draughts. Baby clothing needs frequent washing and it is best to avoid using detergents for this as they are liable to irritate the delicate skin.

Bathing. At first a baby is bathed once a day, usually in the morning before his mid-morning feed. Later on when he is more active he usually needs an evening wash as well as a morning bath. For a baby's bath the room must be warm and free from draughts. Everything likely to be needed must be put ready and clothing put to warm.

The temperature of the water should be about 40°C (approximately 100°F). It must always be tested with a bath thermometer and well mixed. The cold water should be put in the bath first and the hot added.

Requirements. These are as follows:

Two soft towels.
Superfatted soap.
Petroleum jelly.
Disposable napkins.
Safety pins (which must always be kept closed).
Clean clothing.

The tray for swabbing the eyes should contain the following:

Sterile water.
Sterile swabs.
Disposal bag or receiver for used swabs.

The nurse should wear a mackintosh apron and tuck a towel round her waist—for tiny babies she should wear a mask and gown—and first she should wash her own hands.

Procedure: The procedure is as follows:

(1) Swab the baby's eyes, using each swab once only and swabbing from the inner to the outer corner.

(2) Swab and dry the face without using soap.

(3) Wash and dry the hair, holding the baby under his left arm over the bath, with your hand supporting his head.

(4) With the baby lying on your knee lather his body with soap, then, putting your left arm under the baby's head and back, grasping his left arm with your left hand and holding his legs with your other hand, lower him gently into the bath.

(5) After splashing him with water to remove the soap and allowing him to kick and exercise his legs, lift him onto your lap, wrap him in a towel and pat him dry. Care should be taken to see that all creases and folds are quite dry. A little powder may be dusted into folds, but care should be taken to see that only a little is used. Petroleum jelly may be applied to the buttocks.

(6) If the baby is only a few days old and the stump of the umbilical cord has not separated, powder is applied to this and it is covered with a dressing held in place by a crêpe bandage taped to secure.

(7) Next the baby's vest and napkin are put on and finally the clothes drawn on over the feet.

The baby should wear a warm nightgown but must not be overloaded with bedclothes. Soiled linen should be removed at once and the bath and equipment cleared away.

Feeding. Human milk is the best food for the normal infant. It is at the correct temperature, contains no micro-organisms and has in it special substances which protect the infant from infection. Breast-feeding is ideal because of these things and because it brings mother and child into close contact, so giving the baby that sense of security and love that is his greatest need. The nurse should make sure that the nipple is well in the baby's mouth, that he can breathe and does not have his nose buried in his mother's breast and also that he is swallowing the milk.

When human milk is insufficient or unobtainable *cow's milk* may be given instead. A number of proprietary preparations are available for mothers who cannot feed their babies themselves. Typical reasons for this are inadequate milk production or inverted nipples if the inversion cannot be corrected.

Mothers should be told to seek the advice of the midwife, health visitor or general practitioner who will know the current recommendations. One of the most important factors to be remembered when bottle feeding a baby is the sterility of the feeding bottle, the equipment and the feed.

In backward societies, the value of sterilization is rarely appreciated and it is commonly found that babies become seriously ill because their feeds have been mixed with contaminated water.

Babies are fed either three- or four-hourly up to the age of six months, and it can safely be assumed that the quantity is correct when the child increases in weight normally, is content, does not vomit and has healthy stools. Some people like babies to be fed 'on demand', when they cry and appear to be hungry. This seems to work well.

In a hospital before preparing any feed a nurse must put on a mask and wash her hands. Everything she uses must be sterilized. All the ingredients must be carefully measured.

During feeding the child is, wherever possible, held in the nurse's arms with his head and back supported. The feed should be given slowly, taking about ten to twenty minutes. The teat should be kept full so that air will not be swallowed. The baby should be held up against the nurse's shoulder halfway through the feed so that any wind can be brought up and the bottle may be kept warm by putting it in a jug of warm water. The contents of an unfinished bottle must be thrown away, after the amount has been measured and noted.

A baby needs to be loved, to be held close and cuddled. Caressing and playing with a baby is a vital part of his nursing care and the nurse should always find time for this after each feed. No baby should ever have to take his feed alone with the bottle propped up beside him; the baby could regurgitate and drown without anyone noticing.

Babies' bottles should be rinsed in cold water after use and washed thoroughly in warm water with detergent, using a bottle brush to ensure that all milk is removed. They may be left to sterilize in a solution of Milton 1:80.

Teats must be rubbed with salt to remove the slime from the milk, turned and rinsed well, boiled for two minutes and then stored in a covered jar. Bottles and teats should be boiled once a day. Each baby should have its own bottle and teats and these must be labelled to avoid any baby being given those used by another one.

Health Supervision

From the second week of its life each baby's welfare is supervised by a member of the community health team, the health visitor, who visits and advises the mother. She carries out regular checks on his progress at the Infant Welfare Clinic and provides for immunization when the right time comes. Usually that against poliomyelitis and whooping cough is advised and sometimes against measles as well.

Care of the Sick Child

Today there is a tendency to nurse sick children in their own homes wherever possible rather than in hospital. There are two main reasons for this: (a) it is better for the child not to be separated from his mother and the home environment and (b) there is always the danger of picking up an infection in hospital however much care is taken to prevent this. Many areas now have among the home nursing team nurses who are trained in the nursing of sick children to make care of the child in the home possible.

When a sick child has to be treated in hospital, e.g. for an operation, the nurse must appreciate his special needs and do her best to supply them.

The nurse should never lie to a child. She need not go to the full truth in all its details, but it should never be necessary to tell a lie. Once he finds that a nurse has not told the truth he will not trust her again. She has added to his anxiety and to that extent has delayed his recovery.

If some treatment is going to hurt he should be told. 'You'll feel a sharp prick and then it will all be finished' or 'It stings a bit, but it only lasts a minute', or 'It doesn't really hurt, but it feels a bit funny'. Then he knows what to expect.

If the child must be held while a procedure is carried out, the nurse should do it firmly but kindly as well. Explain simply and quietly what has to be done and that it will help to make him better. The more the child has learnt to trust the nurse the more co-operation he will give.

Admission

When admitting a child the nurse needs the usual information about his name, age and address. In addition, if the patient is a baby the nurse should ask the mother the type of feed he is having, how frequently he is fed, his weight and progress, whether he has been vaccinated or immunized, if he has been baptized and whether he has had any infectious diseases or been in contact with any. If the baby is breast-fed, special arrangements should be made for the mother to continue this at the hospital.

With toddlers and older children the nurse should find out what he calls his potty or what he says when he wants to go to the lavatory. This is most important because some children are desperately shy. Hospital is no place for putting them through the anxiety of learning new ways. The sick child needs all the security he can get and one way of helping him is to use the familiar words and phrases that he has been taught at home. The nurse should enquire about his bed-time routine. If she remembers her own childhood the nurse will know the sort of things to ask. Is he afraid of the dark? Does he have a favourite object that he likes to take to bed? If there is a rhyme to be said, a goodnight phrase to be exchanged, or a prayer? The child's mother should be allowed to stay as long as she can and to help with the routine of temperature taking, getting undressed, bathing and going to bed. He may meet some of the other children while she is still there to give him confidence. A happy child makes a better recovery than a miserable one. Anything the nurse can do to lessen his fears is good nursing.

Settling down

Making use of the information she has gained the nurse can help the child to feel at home in the ward, talking to him of his brothers and sisters, his hobbies, his schoolmates (if he is old enough to go to school), the holidays; all the things that are familiar to him. She can be the link between the hospital and home and must remember to share her information with the other nurses so that they can help him too.

Observation

A child may suffer from many of the diseases that adults do but because of his more delicately balanced nervous system and smaller body he reacts much more quickly to his environment and in a very short time, trifling causes may produce grave symptoms, such as a dramatic rise in temperature, but have apparently no symptoms of disease. He may be gravely ill. For this reason a nurse must be on the alert to notice any change in a child's condition and must exercise great care in taking the temperature, pulse and respiration.

Children are unable to stand a period of starvation before operation, so the surgeon usually orders them to have glucose or barley sugar. After the operation is over the nurse must keep careful watch on the child and record his temperature, pulse and respirations more frequently than is necessary in the case of an adult.

Much can be learned from the cry of a child. A normal cry is loud and strong and the child gets red in the face. A feeble wail or fretful whine indicate pain and exhaustion. A shrill, piercing cry is often a symptom of brain disease. A hoarse, throaty cry indicates laryngitis while loud crying with movements of the arms and legs denotes hunger or a sudden attack of pain.

Bowel movements should be observed very carefully and if abnormal stools are seen the doctor should be informed. At first an infant passes unformed dark greenish-black stools, then the colour becomes yellow and the consistency of scrambled eggs. It does not become brown and formed until starch is included in the diet. Frequent small dark green stools in an older baby are an indication that the baby is not having enough feeds, while large green ones prove, as do bulky ones, that a baby is being overfed. Hard crumbly, stools are a sign of constipation. Pale stools may be a sign of serious disorder and should be reported to the doctor. Fat in the stools may mean pancreatic disorder while the presence of curds proves that the feed is not being digested and needs diluting. A grey, alkaline, offensive, crumbly stool is a proof that the feed contains too much protein, while an unformed, yellowish brown frothy acid one means too much sugar.

Visiting

Children cannot be reasoned with like adults. The younger the child the harder is is for him to understand why his mother has to leave him just at the time that he needs her most of all. The bewilderment and unhappiness he goes through at this time may have a permanent effect on his emotional development.

It is now recognized that all children in hospital should be visited as frequently and for as long as possible and that the mothers of children under five should be with their children all the time. Many hospitals today have special accommodation for mothers so that they can come in with their children and stay with them during their time in hospital. If a mother cannot stay—perhaps she has other small children to care for at home—she should be allowed to visit whenever she likes and for as long as she can manage. Most hospitals are doing this, but some still insist on fixed visiting hours.

Nurses sometimes wonder whether it is good for a child to be visited because he cries when his mother has to go away again. Studies have shown that it is better for a child to be visited, even if he cries after each visit, than that he should be 'good' and unvisited. The child who cries can be comforted and he soon learns that his mother will come back. The quiet child is keeping all his grief to himself and may think his mother has abandoned him, the most dreadful thing that can happen in a child's world. A quiet child is a sick child, either physically or emotionally, or both.

Ward routine

Because the healthy child is noisy, active and adventurous, a children's ward cannot be run quite like one for adults. Beds will be untidy, toys will be strewn about, children as they get better will be in and out of bed. Although a certain amount of law and order is necessary for everyone's peace of mind, the nurse should let the children have as much freedom as possible. The school teacher and the occupational therapist will keep them interested and occupied for part of the day and hospitals which allow open visiting find that parents are a great help, not only in playing with the children but at mealtimes and bedtime too. They help with the routine feeding and washing, leaving the nurse more time for special treatments.

The study of sick children is a very specialized one and this section touches only the fringe of the subject. Its object is simply to point out some of the ways the nursing of children differs from that of adults. Imagination and understanding are part of good nursing in every ward, but especially so in the children's ward, because the sick child is so vulnerable.

Adolescents

Adolescents should ideally be nursed in a separate unit suited to their needs and with adequate dayrooms including somewhere where they can continue their studies if they are in hospital for any length of time. They need to be handled firmly but with kindness and tolerance and with understanding of their special problems.

18

Nursing Care of the Elderly

Today, as a result of social improvements and medical advances, many people are living to become old. Ideally old people should have the support of a loving family around them, but, because so many married women go out to work it is becoming increasingly difficult for the old who are too frail to look after themselves to be cared for adequately by their grown-up families.

Many elderly people who are not frail can look after themselves in their own homes, sometimes with help from local social agencies (Meals on Wheels, supervision by the health visitor, or domestic assistance from a home help). Too many are lonely and feel unwanted and shut off from the world, though valuable work is done in some areas by voluntary and church workers who visit old people regularly.

Most old people have lived good and useful lives, have reared families and sent them out into the world, have fought for their country, or in other ways have given of their best for many years. They should not be allowed to feel helpless or a burden to others, with existence becoming a misery as they lose their faculties and strength, but should be given respect for their previous achievements and present knowledge and wisdom.

The changes that take place in old age are common to all. They include impairment of memory for recent events, the tendency to live in the past and to recount the same story over and over again, self-centredness, apparent greed, a desire for sweet things and the demanding of personal attention. It must be remembered that the mental degeneration is brought about by the increasing handicap of an ageing body, the slowing of the circulation, the hardening of the arteries and the degeneration of the brain cells. In addition many have the burden of an accumulation of minor ailments.

Many old people live alone, perhaps in one room which can be reached only by a flight of stairs, so they go out as little as possible. Cooking is a burden, so they live on bread and jam, biscuits, tinned food and cups of tea. They do not take enough protein, vitamins and minerals and become permanently tired and unwell.

Such people can have the services of a home help, who is employed by the Social Services Department of the Local Authority, to do the domestic routines, such as cleaning, cooking, washing and shopping for people who through age or illness cannot do them for themselves. A card may be provided to be put in the window in case of emergency, when help is needed. Other services sometimes available include cheap bus fares, Darby and Joan clubs, holidays and outings and lunch clubs.

Illness in Old Age

The kinds of illness which affect the older patients are those which come from the ageing of their bodies and the changes which take place in their tissues, rather than the short, acute conditions of younger people. The branch of medicine and nursing which deals with the care of the aged is called geriatrics. The illnesses from which old people suffer include:

(1) Heart disease, leading to congestive heart failure.
(2) Carcinoma (cancer) spreading usually more slowly than in younger people.
(3) Cerebral arteriosclerosis with haemorrhage or thrombosis resulting in hemiplegia (stroke).
(4) Arthritis.
(5) Parkinson's disease.
(6) Chronic bronchitis, particularly in smokers.
(7) Fractures, especially of the neck of the femur, because old people may be unsteady and their bones are brittle.
(8) Senility with resulting mental changes, and leading to general bodily neglect and undernourishment.

The complications in all illness which good nursing aims to prevent are:

(1) Pressure sores due to lying too long in one position or to the sodden skin associated with incontinence.
(2) Retention of urine and infection of the bladder.
(3) Constipation.
(4) Stiff joints and contractures due to leaving limbs too long in one position without exercising them.

(5) Malnutrition because the patient may have very little appetite or be faddy about food offered.

(6) Pneumonia caused by poor circulation and lack of movement.

Care of the Elderly Patient in Hospital

There is a spirit of optimism today about the care of elderly patients in hospitals. After a preliminary assessment many are found to be suitable for rehabilitation and return home.

A great deal is being done today for old people by physical medicine. The bedridden are taught to walk again, the crippled to do for themselves many things that were impossible a few years ago. Nobody is too old today for successful treatment, but the most valued ally that geriatric medicine has is a team of workers who really understand their old patients, who treat them with dignity and respect and who give them a sense of security and, above all, a sense of being wanted. There is so much they can pass on to younger people from the wisdom which comes from experience. If they do not always seem to be wise, but sometimes obstinate or difficult, the nurses should remember that age brings physical changes to the brain as well as to other tissues. They must be encouraged, never bullied or scolded, to make those movements or perform those tasks that are going to make them still happy members of the community for per- haps several years longer. There is more scope for nursing skill in geriatric nursing than in any other branch and it needs the best of nurses.

Although elderly patients in hospital need the same care as all sick people there are certain points that need special emphasis.

Mobility

All patients should get up as soon as possible, partly because it will prevent pressure sores, muscle wastage and pneumonia but also because if they are encouraged to stay in bed they soon lose the will to get up and their health, both physical and mental, deteriorates rapidly. If a patient cannot get dressed it may be possible to nurse him, for a time, in an armchair with his feet on a footstool. This will allow his lungs to expand more fully and relieve distressed breathing. Various types of hoist in use in hospital wards can lift quite heavy people out of bed and put them in a wheel- or armchair.

Old people are very susceptible to changes in temperature and quickly get chills. As they tend to move slowly they should be warmly and comfortably clad and wear comfortable shoes. Slippers should be avoided because they give no support to the feet and may be the cause of an old person tripping.

When the patient gets up the nurse should see that he has clean handkerchiefs and a bag to hold his precious possessions like spectacles or sweets, before being taken to a dayroom or the occupational therapy department. Not to be able to put his hands on some personal belonging can cause him great distress.

Old people depend a great deal on their feet. Corns, ingrowing toenails, bunions and any other disability which makes walking difficult must be reported at once so that the chiropodist can attend to it. If old people need help when walking they should be supplied with walking sticks of the right length tipped with rubber; a walking frame may be useful.

Floors in a geriatric ward should never be polished and a non-slip plastic finish is generally used. Rugs are dangerous as they may slip and carpets should be inspected frequently for worn or threadbare patches which could cause an accident. Even a slight fall can mean a broken leg for an old person because his bones are so brittle.

Nourishment

Nourishing food, taken regularly, always brings out a surprising improvement in an elderly person's condition.

The nurse should make sure that patients who have dentures use them. If they keep taking them out there is probably something wrong with them. The sister should be informed if this is the case so that they can be attended to.

Meals should be served punctually and as daintily and appetizingly as possible, giving small helpings to begin with and wherever possible, taking note of individual likes and dislikes; some like their food dry, others prefer it moistened. Many people hate using a spoon instead of a knife and fork, even if the spoon is easier to handle.

Bowels

Old people and those suffering from long-term illness do not tolerate strong purgatives and may require suppositories or enemas. The disposable enema is particularly useful here. Instead of a bedpan they should have a commode provided whenever they can use one or be wheeled to the lavatory.

It is worth finding out whether the patient has been in the habit of taking a laxative regularly and what particular brand he has been using. When a habit has been established over a number of years it is not always wise to break it off completely, but much can be done to relieve constipation by including fruit and vegetables and plenty of fluids in the diet and by getting the patient moving. Even if he is unable to get up he should be encouraged to move his legs up and down and to change his position frequently.

Occupation and recreation

Stagnation of any kind leads to decay and unless old people live as regular and normal a life as possible and are provided with stimulating contacts, they deteriorate rapidly both physically and mentally. They should have visitors, newspapers, books and magazines, interesting hobbies and should not be encouraged to think of themselves as chronic invalids. They should be put under care of the occupational therapist as soon as they are well enough.

Apart from physical care old people have two great needs. They need companionship and they need to feel that they still count as individuals. Loneliness and the feeling that no-one would really care if they died tomorrow are often the basic factors which lead to depression, apathy, malnutrition and finally physical illness. The nurse can do much to revive an old person's self esteem and interest in life. She should look for any little way in which to emphasize his individuality. If there is room in the ward for patients to have photographs or small personal belongings on their lockers, she should let them do so and make a point of talking about them whenever she can. She can keep a list of all the birthdays in the ward and make a little celebration of each one. It may be only birthday wishes and telling the other patients, but perhaps the kitchen can provide a birthday cake as well; this is often possible if enough warning is given. Do not be put off if a cake is out of the question because it is the remembering that counts most. Try to keep a little extra jam in store, or a packet of brightly coloured paper table napkins. There is no need to stop at birthdays. Any little happening can be the excuse for a celebration to draw attention to a patient as an individual. 'Mrs Green has walked the full length of the ward today for the first time, let's have a celebration'; 'Mr Black's son has just been promoted to works manager, we've only got tea but all the same we'll drink his health'. If a nurse gets into the habit of thinking this way she will soon have plenty of ideas.

Patients who can get up can play cards, ludo or draughts or watch television. Some of those in bed may be able to do some knitting or crochet, make baskets or read the newspapers. Other may be too frail or disabled to do any of these things. More than anything else they need someone to talk with them. This can be difficult for a nurse in a busy ward, but every time she carries out any nursing care for them she can exchange a few words with them at the same time. So many nurses chatter at patients thinking that they are cheering them up, but the flow of talk goes over the old person's head. He is bemused and cannot take it in, so he makes no response.

Not all old people are deaf, so a nurse should not shout unless it is absolutely necessary. She should keep her voice at the normal level, but get the old person's attention before she starts. When she has said anything to him she should wait for him to answer, although it may be thirty seconds or more before he can get the words out. Two sentences spoken by the patient to a nurse are worth more than any amount of bright talk on her part if he does not respond.

Visitors
Visitors can be the life blood of a geriatric ward. They keep the patient in touch with the outside world, with home and the family, with friends and neighbours. Nurses should do all they can to make visitors feel welcome, learning their names and always using them. If they see a visitor struggling to make conversation with a patient but having no success, they should go and help. In between visits patients should be encouraged to write to their visitors. A short simple note is all that is needed, just to say how much they enjoyed the visit and that they are looking forward to the next. If a patient cannot do this himself the nurse should offer to write for him. Visitors should be valued partners of the nursing staff and the doctor and the ward sister should always be available to see them.

Preparation for going home
Many patients, after assessment and treatment, may soon be able to go home. It is often helpful if visits home for tea or for a longer period, a week-end say, can be arranged so that the patient can become gradually used to being away from the hospital. Before discharge contact should be made with the health visitor, community nurse and social services department of the area where the patient lives, so that supervision and care can be provided.

Day Hospitals

After discharge home old people may be able to attend a day hospital two or three days a week, and while there will be encouraged to take part in social activities, to continue with occupational therapy and to receive physiotherapy or any other treatment that may be needed. These day hospitals are most valuable, not only for the continued care and supervision given, but because they enable old people to get out of their homes and meet others in their age group. One elderly lady who visits one of these day hospitals regularly told her home help, who had noticed that she did not grumble nearly as much as she used to, 'I never realized there were so many people worse off than myself.'

Those people who need to have continuous care in an institution may be able to have this in a hospital near to their homes and families. The increasing number of 'community hospitals' are ideal for this, where the patient can be looked after by his or her own family doctor.

19

The Human Body

We are quite accustomed to hear ourselves spoken of as individuals and this is a very accurate use of the word. Each of us is unlike any other person there has been and unlike anyone born after us. Even our children will be different from us though they may have some of our characteristics; that is to say they will be like one or both parents and the children of one family will resemble each other. But unless they are identical twins they will not be exactly alike.

The cell

The cell is a microscopic and very simple structure. It consists of a jelly-like substance called protoplasm enclosed in a thin pliable cover, the cell membrane. Cell protoplasm is called cytoplasm and in this is a

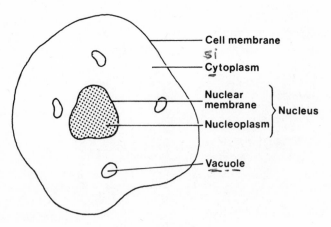

Fig. 7. A typical cell.

darker part called the nucleus which consists of nucleoplasm contained in a nuclear membrane.

In lower life forms reproduction is by fission or splitting. The nucleus splits in two, each part becoming a new complete nucleus. The cell itself then divides to take a new nucleus in each half thereby forming two new cells identical to the original one. In turn the daughter cells divide to form more identical cells and in this way the species reproduces itself. But it only produces more cells of the same form and having the same properties.

Mitosis. In higher forms of life the process is more complex and is called mitosis. The human cell, whether it is a bone cell, a muscle cell or a nerve cell, contains forty-six chromosomes. The chromosomes contain the genes which carry all the information and instructions for succeeding generations of cells. In the embryo, cells develop in different ways so that some make bone, others make blood vessels and others make lungs. The cells become specialized by a process known as differentiation.

In mitosis the forty-six chromosomes in the cell split in two along their length; each half of a chromosome moves away from its other half and when the cell divides the new cells each contain forty-six chromosomes. Mitosis is not reproduction of the species, only reproduction of the cells.

Meiosis is a process in which cells split in a way quite different from mitosis. The chromosomes do not split but half of them, twenty-three, go to one new cell and the other half, twenty-three, go to another daughter cell. These cells are used for reproduction of the species, one from the female and one from the male. When fertilization takes place one male gamete (sperm), as these cells are called, and one female gamete (ovum) fuse together to form a new cell with the full number of chromosomes, forty-six.

Twins. When two or more ova are fertilized at the same time a multiple pregnancy results though the twins are non-identical. Twins developing from one ovum are very similar in appearance and are known as identical twins.

Organs

In the developing embryo cells collect together to form the various organs of the body. An organ is a group of tissues arranged to perform a specific task, e.g. the heart to pump blood or a bone to provide structural strength.

Systems

A system is a grouping of organs which together carry out a special function. There are nine systems as follows:

(1) The skeletal system: structure.

(2) The muscular system: movement.

(3) The respiratory system: oxygen intake, carbon dioxide excretion.

(4) The digestive system: chemical breakdown of food into absorbable substances.

(5) The circulatory system: transport within the body of food, oxygen and waste products.

(6) The excretory system: removal of waste matter.

(7) The reproductive system: reproduction of the species.

(8) The nervous system: internal communication and response to the surroundings.

(9) The endocrine system: manufacture of a wide range of chemicals, some of which have a control function.

These systems are closely interrelated and the faulty function of one will affect the others. The body as a whole can tolerate a fairly severe degree of bad treatment, e.g. undernourishment, loss of blood, excessive heat or fear, though if any of these is continued the compensating mechanisms fail to fulfil their purpose. For example, if the production of digestive fluids is inadequate, food is not broken down into assimilable compounds and in young children growth may be severely impaired. Bad circulation of blood or shallow breathing result in a shortage of oxygen in the tissues and general physical weakness. The miner who as a young man revelled in his strength becomes as a result of inhaling dust for many years, a chronic bronchitic, quite incapable of a day's work; his muscles will not obey his will.

Symptoms and signs of illness

When a physician examines a patient, he listens to what the patient says about pain or discomfort and makes tests of temperature, pulse rate and so on; he does not at once jump to a diagnosis. A healthy looking bronzed skin may indicate Addison's disease, a disease of the adrenal glands. The physician knows that illness in one system will be shown in another—spots on a patient's chest may not be due to an infection but to eating too many strawberries.

Classification of diseases and disorders

Diseases are best considered in groups. Some, such as congenital diseases, are most commonly seen and treated in children. Other conditions such as degenerative diseases are more frequent in the elderly. This is because, mainly owing to medical and social advances, more people are living to old age, more than the biblical age of three score years and ten. The majority of disorders are, however, found in any age group, and are classified as follows:

Infectious diseases are the result of the entry of pathogenic micro-organisms into the body. They can cause either general malaise, or specific identifiable infections such as measles.

Congenital disorders. This group includes diseases or handicaps, both mental and physical, which are present at or before birth. Examples are:

(1) Congenital dislocation of the hip owing to faulty development in the uterus.

(2) Cerebral palsy (spasticity) arising from injury during birth.

Degenerative disorders are associated with the wearing out of tissues usually as the result of advancing years but often accelerated by injury or misuse. Examples are arthritis and arterial degeneration leading to strokes.

Endocrine disorders are illnesses associated with the hormone systems of the body. Imbalance of these hormones causes illness. Examples are thyrotoxicosis which is caused by deficiency of thyroid secretion. Diabetes mellitus is caused by inadequate production of insulin from the pancreas.

Neoplasms otherwise called growths or tumours are the result of uncontrolled multiplication of cells in the body. They can either be benign or malignant.

Benign growths are usually encapsulated and therefore are contained and do not spread to different parts of the body. The main damage they do is due to the exertion of pressure on adjoining tissues. An example is a fibroid growth which presses on the muscle of the uterus.

Malignant growths are not encapsulated but invade other tissues which they then destroy. They are easily spread by the blood stream and lymphatic system causing secondary deposits in other parts of the body. They can also be spread by contact, for example a stomach cancer cell can drop onto and invade another structure in the abdominal cavity.

Behavioural disorders are pathological variations of normal behaviour. They include:

(1) Drug addiction and dependence.
(2) Alcoholism.
(3) Compulsive eating.
(4) Anxiety, depression and suicide.
(5) Obsessional behaviour.
(6) Hallucinations and irrational convictions.

Despite the advances of medicine more and more people are requiring hospital care for these types of disorders.

Trauma. Traumatic injury is injury caused by physical or chemical accidents and is the main cause of death and disablement in young people. Physical trauma can be due to violence such as gunshot wounds, knife wounds, blows or to accidents in the home or on the roads. Chemical trauma is caused by taking poisons into (or onto) the body. They can be taken in the form of solids, liquids or gases and may be taken deliberately or accidentally.

20

Basic Physical Principles

The many and varied processes which take place in the living body are applications of a small number of physical and chemical principles. Your understanding of bodily events will be greatly increased if you know the scientific basis of these processes.

All material is made up of minutely small particles called molecules and is in one of the three states, that is to say solid, liquid or gas. A solid has its own shape, a liquid takes up the shape of its container and a gas completely occupies the space in which it is contained. A liquid will fall to the bottom of its container but a heavy gas like chlorine or a light gas like hydrogen fills the cylinders which contains each of them. Molecules in the liquid or gaseous state are in constant movement and this movement is increased by raising the temperature. If ice is heated it melts to become water which in turn with more heating boils and turns into water vapour. The process is reversed if heat is extracted or lost.

Gas pressure

Molecules are mutually attracted to each other strongly in solids but less so in liquids and gases. The gas in a cylinder of oxygen for example will fill the cylinder evenly and if more gas is forced in, the total amount of gas (at higher pressure) will occupy the whole cylinder. As the gas is used the pressure drops until gas is no longer forced out and a new cylinder must be attached to whatever equipment is being used.

If the pressure of oxygen in the lungs is low it will not be taken up by the blood. This explains why work at high altitudes is harder to carry out and it is the reason for pressurizing aircraft cabins.

Dissolution

Dissolution (dissolving) is the taking up of a substance (liquid, solid or gas) by a liquid to form a solution whose composition is the same throughout. Common salt, sodium chloride, will dissolve in water and though not stirred will in time be evenly distributed. There is a limit to the amount of salt that a certain amount of water will dissolve and a solution which will not dissolve any more is said to be saturated.

Absorption

Absorption occurs when one substance enters the surface of another. For example a bath towel dries the skin by absorbing the water from it and proteins, carbohydrates and fats are absorbed by the walls of the small intestine.

Diffusion

Diffusion is a process of self-mixing of gas with gas, of gas with liquid and of liquid with liquid. It is a result of the agitation of molecules in a gas or, in solution, of the ions.

If two solutions of small molecules are separated by a fine sieve called a semipermeable membrane which allows the passage of small molecules but not of large molecules, total mixing occurs and the amount of solution on either side remains unchanged.

Two gases which do not react chemically will totally intermix. Nitrous oxide and oxygen in equal quantities are premixed in one cylinder and used for analgesia of the mother during labour; the mixture is called Entonox.

Osmosis

Let us now consider the situation when molecules too large to pass through the semipermeable membrane are in solution, sugar in water for instance. The water can pass freely to and fro but the sugar on each side cannot. If the solution on one side is stronger and on the other weak, water will diffuse through to the stronger side until the two solutions are of equal concentration. In other words the stronger solution will increase in volume and the level on its side of the membrane will rise. This process, known as osmosis, is in one direction only and therefore serves as a pump; if more sugar is added to the strong side yet more water will be extracted from the weaker side. It is by this process that tissue fluid is taken from the tissues and enters the veins. In a starving person who lacks plasma protein the tissue fluid is not removed and oedema of starvation ensues. This distressing condition is particularly obvious in starving children and babies whose plump abdomens and faces may give the appearance of overeating.

Filtration

Filtration is the separation of a solid from a liquid by the simple means of pushing the liquid through holes smaller than the suspended particles.

21

Bone

When fully developed, bones consist of about one-third organic matter consisting of cells, blood vessels and a gelatinous substance called collagen—and two-thirds mineral matter comprising calcium and phosphate. In young children the proportion of organic matter is greater so the bones are softer and pliable. Extra minerals are added over the years and in old people the bones are harder but very brittle and thus break easily.

The outer part of a bone is very dense almost like ivory; this is called compact bone. Nearer the middle it is much looser, rather like a

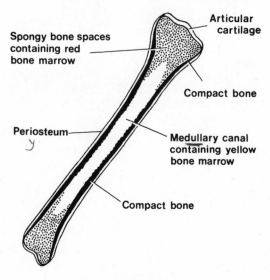

Fig. 8. Bone.

honeycomb and is called cancellous bone. In the middle is a space. This serves not only to reduce the weight of the bone but also holds the bone marrow which manufactures red and white blood cells. In

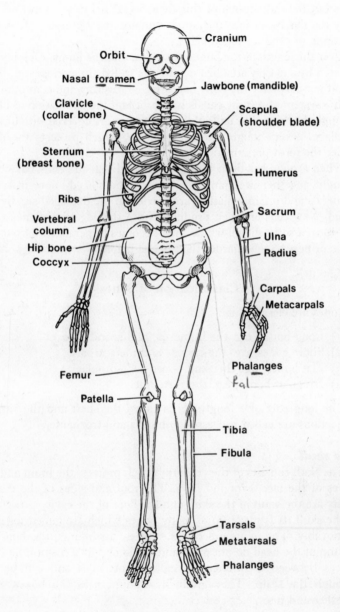

Fig. 9. The human skeleton.

children all the bones have marrow which actively produces blood cells but in adults much of this turns to fat or 'yellow marrow' and only the flat bones and the upper ends of the humerus and femur continue to produce blood cells.

Over the length of the bones, though not at the joints, each bone is covered by a closely attached membrane called the periosteum. Tiny blood vessels pierce the bone beneath this covering and communicate with a system of minute canals which permit the circulation of blood through the bone. The ends of the long bones are covered with hyaline cartilage, a very tough form of cartilage, which protects the parts under the most pressure.

When a bone has been broken, provided that the ends have been brought together well and the limb immobilized, new materials (minerals and organic matter) are carried to the damaged site by the blood. New cells are then produced from the edges until they meet and form a soft callous, which then becomes mineralized. Often this piece of new bone is harder than it was before.

Classification of Bones

Bones are classified as:

(1) Long bones, e.g. the humerus, radius and ulna.
(2) Short bones, e.g. the carpals and metacarpals.
(3) Flat bones, e.g. the skull bones and scapula.
(4) Irregular bones, e.g. the vertebrae.

The long part of a long bone is called the shaft and the various projections are called processes, condyles and trochanters.

The skull

The skull consists of the cranium which protects the brain and the bones of the face, ears and jaws. The roof and sides of the cranial cavity are the vault of the skull and the floor of the cavity is the base of the skull. It is made up of many bones which are joined together immovably. The joints are called sutures. In infants, the bones at the top of the head do not meet and are joined by a membrane. The spaces between the bones are called fontanelles and can be felt through the scalp. They gradually disappear as the bones grow together and fuse.

Sinuses are hollow spaces in the bones of which there are several

sphinx

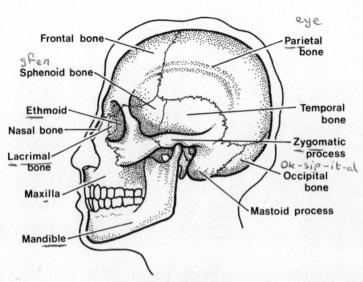

eye

sfen

Ok-sip-it-al

Fig. 10. Side view of the skull.

such spaces in the head. They are filled with air and lined by a mucous membrane which is continuous with that which lines the nose. They give lightness but rigidity to the bones and also tone and resonance to the voice. It is these that may become blocked during colds causing thickening of the voice. The sinuses open into the nose and cause great discomfort if they become inflamed producing the condition called sinusitis.

The chest

The bones of the chest, or thorax are:

(1) The sternum, the flat, dagger-shaped bone in the front of the chest.

(2) The ribs of which there are twelve pairs. They are attached by cartilage to the vertebrae at the back and to the sternum in the front. The exceptions are the bottom two pairs, which are attached only to the vertebrae and so are called 'floating' ribs.

The spine

The spinal column is a flexible structure supporting the head and protecting the spinal cord. It consists of the vertebrae which are separated by the vertebral discs.

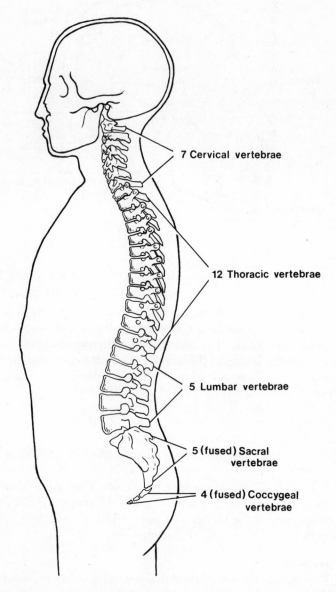

7 Cervical vertebrae

12 Thoracic vertebrae

5 Lumbar vertebrae

5 (fused) Sacral
        vertebrae

4 (fused) Coccygeal
        vertebrae

Fig. 11. The spinal column; note that the lower vertebrae are larger to
support the greater weight.

The vertebrae

There are thirty-three vertebrae. They are divided into:

(1) Seven cervical (neck) vertebrae.

(2) Twelve thoracic (chest) vertebrae.

(3) Five lumbar vertebrae.

(4) Five sacral vertebrae which are fused in adults forming the sacrum.

(5) Four coccygeal (pronounced *coxigeal*) vertebrae which are fused in adults to form the coccyx.

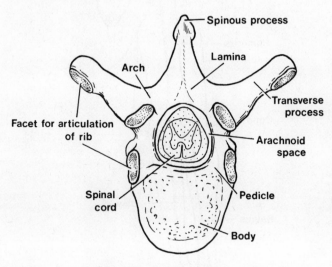

Fig. 12. A simple vertebra.

A vertebra consists of the body, the arch and several processes, two of which are attached to the ribs; others control the flexibility of the spine. The arch surrounds the canal which holds the spinal cord.

Invertebral discs

Between the bodies of the vertebrae are discs of cartilage which act as buffers in absorbing sudden pressure. They also aid freedom of movement. If one of these discs is bruised or damaged it can press on surrounding tissue and cause pain and backache. This condition is commonly (and inaccurately) known as a 'slipped disc'. The discs separate the vertebrae and allow a limited amount of rotation.

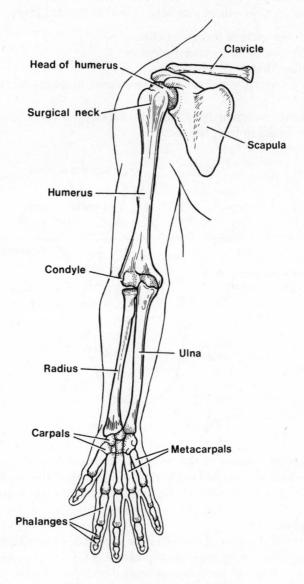

Fig. 13. Upper limb and shoulder.

The shoulder-girdle

The shoulder-girdle provides suspension for the arms. It consists of a clavicle (collar bone) and scapula on each side. The clavicle is a long bone with a double curve and lies above the first rib, articulating with the sternum and scapula. The scapula is a large flat triangular bone on the back of each shoulder.

The bones of the upper limb

The humerus is a long bone with a head which fits into a shallow cup on the scapula. The lower end has two condyles where it meets the two long bones of the forearm. The upper part of the shaft is sometimes called the surgical neck as it is so easily broken.

The forearm consists of two bones, the radius and the ulna. They are designed to give the remarkable rotating quality of the forearm.

The radius is on the 'thumb' side of the arm. The pulse is most easily taken at the point where the radial artery passes over the top of this bone in the wrist. The ulna is on the little finger side of the arm and its upper end forms the prominence of the elbow.

The eight carpals are small irregularly shaped bones in the wrist. The five metacarpals form the palm of the hands. Each finger is made up of three phalanges and the thumb of two phalanges. The thumb has been separated from the fingers during the course of evolution until, as now, it can be moved opposite the fingers to grasp objects.

The pelvis

The pelvis consists of the hip-bone, the sacrum and the coccyx.

The hip-bone consists of three fused bones—the ilium, ischium and pubis. The ilium is the broad part of the hip, the ischium is the lower part which one sits with and the pubic is the bone which can be felt at the front of one's hips. Together the bones are called the innominate bones, but this term is not used much.

The socket which holds the head of the femur is called the acetabulum and is formed of all three bones fused together.

A woman's pelvis is wider than a man's and the inside cavity larger and more circular as it has to allow delivery of a baby.

The bones of the lower limb

In medical terminology the word 'leg' refers only to the part between the knee and the ankle. The upper part of the limb is always referred to as the thigh.

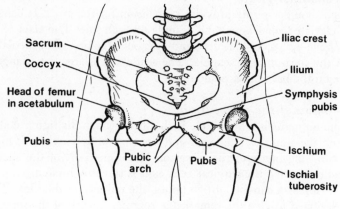

Sacrum
Coccyx
Head of femur in acetabulum
Pubis
Pubic arch
Pubis
Iliac crest
Ilium
Symphysis pubis
Ischium
Ischial tuberosity

Fig. 14. The pelvis.

The femur, or thigh bone, is the longest, strongest and heaviest bone in the body. Its head fits into the acetabulum and forms the hip-joint. The shaft ends in two bony condyles at the knee. These condyles articulate with the tibia and fibula. The tibia is the inner bone of the leg; it has a sharp ridge at the bottom which is the shin. The fibula is the outer bone of the leg and articulates with the tibia at its upper end. The two bones are arranged like a brooch with its pin.

The bones of the foot consist of seven tarsals, five metatarsals and the fourteen phalanges in the toes which are similar to those in the fingers.

The arches of the foot

The arches of the foot support the weight of the body. The arches are formed by:

(1) The shape and arrangement of the bones.
(2) The tension of the ligaments.
(3) The muscle and fasciae in the sole of the foot.

There are two longitudinal arches and one transverse arch. Sometimes these arches drop and the feet ache badly producing the condition called flat-foot. It is produced by certain weakening illnesses, by jobs that involve a great deal of walking or standing, or by wearing badly designed shoes. The foot should always point forwards, and

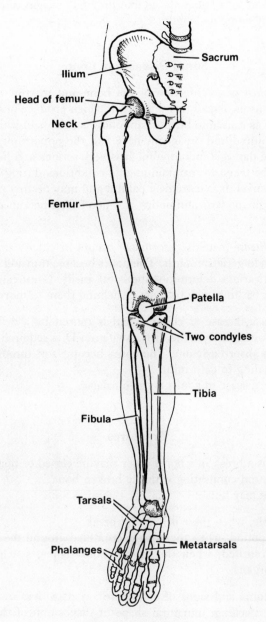

Fig. 15. Lower limb.

not allowed to turn outwards, so that the body weight can be distributed evenly along its length.

Some Diseases of Bone

Osteomyelitis is an infection of the bone and marrow caused by micro-organisms, usually staphylococci, which produce pus. It is not as common as it used to be, but can follow accidents in which a bone has been injured and organisms have had the opportunity to enter through the damaged periosteum. It is very serious and hence great care must be taken to maintain aseptic conditions during bone surgery. Osteomyelitis is extremely painful and may destroy part of the bone, though modern antibiotics and good nursing can cure most cases.

Paget's disease (osteitis deformans) occurs in elderly people, and may be seen in geriatric wards. The bones become thin and extremely brittle with various deformities and break easily. Great care must be taken when bathing such patients or helping them to move.

Rickets is a disease of children and is caused by a deficiency of calcium or vitamin D in the diet, as vitamin D is required to enable the body to absorb calcium. The bones become soft through lack of calcium, leading to deformities.

A similar disease in adults is osteomalacia.

Fractures

A fracture is a break in a bone. They may be closed or there may be an open wound connecting with the broken bone.

Fractures may be:

(1) Simple, when there is a 'clean' break.

(2) Compound, when the bone is crumbled around the break.

(3) Complicated, when the broken bone damages neighbouring tissues or organs.

The symptoms and signs of a fracture are pain, loss of voluntary movement, swelling, unnatural shape or disposition of the limb or body and shock.

First aid treatment for fractures:

(1) Assess the situation.

(2) Send at once for an ambulance.

(3) See that the patient can breathe.

(4) Stop any bleeding and cover any broken skin with a very clean dressing, but bleeding from the ears should not be stopped as otherwise pressure might build up in the brain.

(5) Reassure the patient.

(6) Do not move the patient: it is better to leave a person lying in the road and divert the traffic.

(7) Do not move the limb: this is a job for the expert.

(8) Never do more than is absolutely necessary.

An injured motor-cyclist who walked out of a hospital completely well, had been found lying almost in a circle. He owes his life to the ambulance men who got him to hospital without changing his position by an inch. On the other hand, a woman who had a simple fracture of one of the cervical bones died because a well-meaning onlooker slipped a cushion under her head.

Care of a patient with a fracture

When a patient sustains a fractured bone it is accompanied by considerable pain, swelling and loss of movement of the limb which may lie in an unnatural position. These local effects of the fracture will be associated with the general reaction of shock which manifests itself with an ashen pallor, cold clammy skin, rapid pulse and a low blood pressure. The limb must be immobilized to prevent further damage and the patient confined to bed to counteract the shock. Analgesics may be ordered to relieve the pain.

Local immobilization can be achieved by the use of splints, bandages or sandbags or by the application of plaster of Paris. Sometimes a limb is put in traction so that it is properly extended.

The patient should be observed regularly and, at least to begin with, observations should be made half-hourly. These should include pulse, blood pressure and the condition of the injured area.

Once the patient has been treated for shock and his blood pressure is satisfactory, he will, if it is necessary, be prepared for surgery to reduce the fracture. This means putting the bones back in their correct position. Once this has been done the position can be maintained either by inserting metal pins into the bones or covering the limb with plaster of Paris.

While the plaster of Paris is drying, the bedding should be protected by polythene or mackintosh sheets and plenty of air should be allowed to circulate around the plaster to speed up the drying process. A helpful way to achieve this, is to put a bed cradle over the plaster and turn the bedclothes back over it. However, direct heat should not be applied as quick drying of the plaster can make it crack and the heat can cause irritation to the skin underneath. The plaster should be examined regularly and the limb watched to see that it does not become cold, numb, discoloured or painful. It is very important to detect any local areas of plaster pressure and areas which have become overheated.

Nursing care aims to prevent respiratory infections and so the patient must be sat up after regaining consciousness. Urinary infection can be prevented by ensuring that the patient has plenty to drink. Venous thrombosis and stiffness of joints is prevented by physiotherapy and bed sores can be prevented by turning the patient regularly and frequently and encouraging him to move his good limbs. He is allowed to get out of bed as soon as is possible. Diet should be rich in protein, calcium and vitamins C and D to promote growth of new bone and healing of surrounding tissues.

Patients admitted to hospital with fractures tend to be in hospital for a long time, so the atmosphere should be homely but well organized. Many patients are young adults suffering from sporting or motor-cycle injuries. The other large group of patients are the elderly as their bones are brittle and they are more liable than most people to fall over. It is essential that they be made to feel happy and at home in their new surroundings. If not, they are liable to become confused and distressed, particularly at night.

22

Muscles and Joints

The function of muscle is to cause movement, either deliberately as in walking, or as part of a process we cannot control such as the beating of the heart. Muscles we control are called voluntary muscles, those we do not control are called involuntary; both types work by becoming shorter and fatter. They are always grouped round joints in pairs so that the action at the joint can be reversed. At the elbow the arm bends when the biceps muscle on the front of the upper arm contracts and you can see the biceps fattening. To straighten the arm the triceps muscle at the back of the upper arm contracts and the biceps relaxes; you can feel the biceps going soft and the triceps hardening.

You can also feel your muscles hardening when they make an effort and this shows that they are working even if no movement occurs and they have not in fact shortened.

Most of what you see as a human body is muscle covered by skin; the meat we eat, steak, chops or a leg of lamb is muscle. In addition to providing movement and support the muscles give protection to the main blood vessels which are deep within the limbs and to the vulnerable organs within the trunk.

The heart is a special muscular organ; one of the most powerful is the uterus which consists of bands of muscle arranged in a criss-cross pattern to expel the fetus at birth.

Muscles

Voluntary muscles

Voluntary muscles are attached to bone by tendons. The energy which enables muscles to work comes from the burning up of food-stuffs, mainly carbohydrates, from which glucose, the main fuel of the body, is produced. Muscular activity is the result of a very complicated series of chemical reactions for which glucose and oxygen, both of which are brought to the muscles in the blood stream, are essential. Muscular effort is therefore dependent upon adequate food supply and a good circulation.

The muscles of the face are responsible for movements of the eyelids, eyebrows, lips and cheeks and for facial expression, speech and mastication.

The skull is covered with a sheet of muscle which is attached to the occipital bone and is inserted into the tissues above the eyebrows, lifting the forehead and drawing the scalp backwards.

The eye has six muscles which provide the very exact movements of the eyeball. The deltoid muscle lies over the shoulder and abducts the arm away from the body; it can be used as a site for giving small intramuscular injections.

The skilled movements of the hand are performed by twenty-seven bones and twenty-eight muscles. The muscles that bend the fingers are called flexors and those that straighten them, extensors.

The diaphragm is the dome-shaped muscle which divides the chest from the abdomen. On breathing in it contracts and lowers, enlarging the chest easily so that more air is taken in. On breathing out it relaxes and assumes its original dome-shape and helps to push air out of the chest. The diaphragm is one of the most important muscles in the body. When it is paralysed, as for example in polio-myelitis, the patient needs a respirator to enable him to breathe. The diaphragm is involved in coughing and hiccups. It also is very important in actions requiring downward pressure, such as defaecating and urinating and in childbirth.

The buttocks are formed by a pair of very strong muscles called the gluteus maximus muscles. They enable us to stand upright, to run and to walk. They are a safe site for intramuscular injections, but care must be taken to avoid the sciatic nerve, which runs underneath the gluteus maximus muscle, by inserting the needle into the upper and outer quadrant of the buttock. In front of the thigh is a big four-part muscle called the quadriceps, which straightens the knee. It also is a safe site for injections. Down the back of the thigh run the hamstrings, which bend the knee. The body is raised on the toes by the action of the gastrocnemius muscle of the calf, which is inserted behind the ankle joint into the point of the heel.

Involuntary muscles

These are found in organs such as the skin, intestine, stomach, bladder and uterus, and are not under the control of the will. They tend to produce different usually rhythmic, movements unlike the voluntary muscles. These movements include:

(1) Peristaltic movements of the intestines.

(2) The beating of the heart.

(3) Raising of the hair follicles of the skin producing the effect of goose pimples.

The involuntary muscles go on working even when we are asleep or unconscious.

Disorders of the muscular system

Fibrositis is what we sometimes think of as rheumatism. It is inflammation of the connective tissue around the muscles and joints. Heat, massage and exercise help to relieve the discomfort.

Muscular dystrophy and myasthenia gravis are serious diseases in which the voluntary muscles gradually lose their power until the patient is absolutely helpless.

The Joints

The chief kinds of joint

These are as follows:

Fibrous or immovable joints. The bones of the skull are locked together in immovable joints known as *sutures.*

Cartilaginous or slightly movable joints. The most common type of slightly movable joint is found in the backbone, where there is sufficient movement between the vertebrae to allow flexion of the spine but not rotation between individual bones. The vertebrae are separated by pads of cartilage.

Synovial or freely-movable joints. The ends of the long bones are thickly covered with articular cartilage. The whole joint is surrounded by a capsule of ligaments and lined by a synovial membrane which secretes synovial fluid. The synovial fluid lubricates the joint so that it moves easily. The ligaments bind the bones together so that they move in the proper direction. A sprain, which is a tear in a ligament, sometimes occurs when a joint is twisted or wrenched. If the joint is torn out of its proper position another form of injury, a dislocation, occurs. There are several types of freely-movable joints, of which the main kinds are:

(1) The ball and socket joint, where a head fits into a cup-shaped socket, e.g. the shoulder and hip.

(2) The pivot joint, where one bone turns on another, e.g. the radius on the ulna when the wrist is rotated.

(3) The hinge joint, where a limb is able to bend in one direction only, e.g. the elbow, the knee and the fingers.

(4) The gliding joint, where the surface of one bone moves over the surface of another, e.g. the bones of the foot.

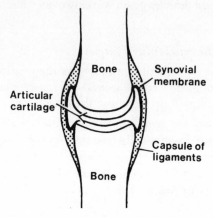

Fig. 16. A freely-movable joint.

Certain definite movements take place at joints and it is useful to know the names of these. They are:

(1) Flexion or bending.
(2) Extension or straightening.
(3) Adduction or movement towards the middle line of the body.
(4) Abduction, movement away from the middle line.
(5) Circumduction, movement of the limb in a circle.
(6) External rotation, turning outward from the middle line.
(7) Internal rotation, turning inward towards the middle line.
(8) Supination, turning the palm of the hand to face upwards.
(9) Pronation or turning the palm downwards.

The best way to learn what these terms mean is to practise the movements with one's own body.

The bones in the principal joints of the body
These are as follows:

(1) The shoulder: scapula (shoulder-blade) and humerus.

(2) The elbow: humerus, radius and ulna.
(3) The wrist: radius and three carpal bones.
(4) The hip: innominate bone and femur.
(5) The knee: femur, tibia and patella (kneecap).
(6) The ankle: tibia, femur and talus.

Some disorders of joints

Acute rheumatism (*rheumatic fever*) is a disease of young people, being more common in hot countries. It can lead to heart disease in later life. There is a fever and the joints, one after another, become very tender, red and swollen. The patient feels, and is, extremely ill and needs extremely skilled and gentle nursing to prevent the heart from becoming affected.

Arthritis is inflammation of the joints.

Rheumatoid arthritis often affects quite young people and recurs in episodes throughout life. It is a crippling and painful condition and is associated with general malaise. The drug cortisone helps to control it, as do other anti-inflammatory agents, but there is no real cure.

Osteo-arthritis usually occurs in later life, the ends of the bones in the joints become rough and any movement hurts. One form of treatment is to operate on the joint and plastic or metal components are often substituted for the bone that is removed.

Bursitis is inflammation of a bursa, that is, one of the sacs filled with synovial fluid situated between the movable parts of a joint. Prepatellar bursitis is called 'housemaid's knee'.

23

The Respiratory System

Respiration, the act of breathing, is the means by which the blood obtains the oxygen which every cell in the body needs. Without oxygen we cannot live for more than a few minutes and if the flow of blood ceases, the brain will suffer irreparable damage in about four minutes.

The control centre of breathing is in the brain stem. When the concentration of carbon dioxide in the blood in the great arteries reaches a certain level, impulses are carried by the vagus and glosso-pharyngeal nerves to the respiratory centre, thence by the phrenic nerves to the diaphragm and by the intercostal nerves to the inter-costal muscles. The muscles then contract and inhalation takes place. This process continues steadily when we are at rest but the rate increases when the physical demands of exercise call for a higher rate of oxygen intake. If the rate of oxygen consumption exceeds the rate of uptake, as in sprinting, the runner becomes exhausted and will slow down however determined he may be to continue. This is why long distances are run very much more slowly; the extra amount of oxygen required by the muscles can be met by deeper or faster breathing. In sprinting no amount of deep breathing can make up for the deficit.

Anatomy

The respiratory tract consists of the nose, the pharynx, the larynx and the trachea. The trachea divides into two passages, the bronchi, one to each lung, which further divide into bronchioles. These in turn subdivide into smaller passages, called alveolar ducts, which lead to the alveoli. The blood system capillaries and respiratory system meet at the alveoli and it is here that oxygen is absorbed into the blood and carbon dioxide taken from it.

The nose which is also the organ of smell has a triangular framework of bone and cartilage covered externally by skin and lined internally with mucous membrane. Hairs in the nostrils filter particles of dust and the stickiness of the mucous membrane traps finer particles and micro-organisms. Blood capillaries serve to warm the inhaled air. Behind the nose lies the nasopharynx which connects the nasal passages to the pharynx below. A further barrier to infection is provided by the adenoids which lies on the posterior surface of the nasopharynx, and the tonsils.

The pharynx lies behind the mouth and is open to it and to the nasopharynx; food or air can pass down it.

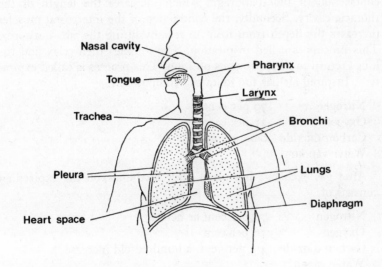

Fig. 17. The respiratory tract.

The larynx starts at the point where the respiratory and alimentary tracts diverge. Its entrance is protected by a leaf-shaped piece of cartilage called the epiglottis which closes during swallowing so as to prevent food or drink entering the larynx. If food does get past it into the larynx we choke, and a sudden cough during swallowing will sometimes force food into the nasal passage. The vocal cords which are essential to speaking or singing are situated in the larynx.

The trachea or windpipe is a tube reaching down into the lungs. Its patency is maintained by incomplete rings of hyaline cartilage and its walls consist of involuntary muscle and fibrous tissue.

The lungs are two conical spongy masses contained each in a separate serous membrane called the pleura. The pleura around each lung is reflected back to line the chest wall, the potential space between the two layers of pleura being the pleural cavity. The outer and inner layers are called the parietal and visceral layers respectively. A little serous fluid between the layers acts as a lubricant to prevent friction.

Respiration

This is a two part process. Firstly, air is sucked into the lungs by the contraction of the diaphragm which increases the length of the thoracic cavity. Secondly, the contraction of the intercostal muscles increases the depth from front to rear by lifting the ribs outwards. This process is called inspiration. The muscles then relax and the lungs return to their previous position. This process is called expiration. Inspired air has the following composition:

Nitrogen	79 per cent
Oxygen	21 per cent
Carbon dioxide	0·04 per cent
Water vapour	

After gas exchange has taken place at the alveoli the expired air consists of:

Nitrogen	79 per cent as before
Oxygen	16 per cent
Carbon dioxide	4·5 per cent, a hundredfold increase
Water vapour	

The breath contains more vapour than the inhaled air does and is one of the ways in which the body excretes water, 400 out of 2600 ml per day. The gas exchange which takes place in the lungs is called external respiration even though it takes place well inside the body. Exchange occurring in the tissues is known as internal respiration.

Respiration is one of the three observations made every day by the nurse, the others being temperature and pulse. The normal rate of respiration is between sixteen and twenty times a minute and because it is not controlled entirely involuntarily, the nurse should disguise the fact that she is timing it, by for example doing so while appearing to count the pulse. She also observes whether it is deep or shallow, irregular, noisy or painful to the patient.

Respiratory distress

The patient who has difficulty with breathing is always fully aware of his condition because shortage of oxygen makes itself very obvious. The cause of breathlessness may be injury to the rib cage, pollution by a toxic gas, shortage of oxygen in the air, or impairment of the breathing reflex arising from trauma of the central nervous system. Respiratory distress is also a common sequel of cardiac failure. Whatever the cause, treatment is directed to re-establishing the exchange of oxygen in the tissues.

Care of the Breathless Patient

All exertion demands the intake of extra oxygen and the patient must not exert himself in any way. Therefore the nurse should do everything possible for her patient. A breathless patient can be very frightened.

Position. In the sitting position the abdominal contents fall away from the lungs and therefore remove some of the pressure against the base of them. This position may be varied by allowing the patient to lean forward in the orthopnoeic position onto a pillow placed on a bed table in front of him. A lightweight blanket should be put around his shoulders to keep them warm.

Comfort. As the patient is nursed upright a foam-rubber or air ring or sheepskin is used for comfort and to prevent his back becoming sore. A pillow placed under the knees, or a footboard will stop him slipping down the bed and a cradle will take the weight of bedclothes.

General toilet. If his condition allows, the patient may be given a blanket bath though if he is very breathless, this may not be possible. His mouth will become dry if he breathes through it for any length of time and also if he is having oxygen. Mouth care must be carried out frequently, the interval being determined by the patient's condition.

Bladder and bowels. Straining for bowel evacuation is tiring and distressing to the patient. A commode requires less effort than a bedpan and the patient will have to be lifted onto it. Glycerine suppositories help the passage of stools. A urinal may be left in position and changed at regular intervals.

Diet. Food which is easily digested will conserve the patient's energy and mouthfuls should be small enough to make sure that he can swallow between breaths. A nurse will always feed her patient to prevent unnecessary effort on his part and must sit down so that he is not hurried or flustered. His locker with a sputum pot, paper handkerchiefs and water must be within easy reach. Frequent visits to his bedside will reassure him that he is being looked after; he may like to have a bell button extension on the bed near at hand.

Visitors. The number of visitors to the breathless patient must for the patient's sake be limited and they must also be told that the patient cannot be expected to hold a normal conversation.

Trachaeostomy

A trachaeostomy is an opening made from the front of the neck into the trachea. It may be part of a regimen of medical or surgical treatment or an emergency procedure. The opening is kept open by the insertion of a special metal or plastic tube. The reasons for a trachaeostomy are:

(1) To bypass an obstruction in the upper respiratory tract.

(2) To improve ventilation by reducing the amount of dead space, i.e. the part of the tract where no gas exchange occurs.

(3) To facilitate suction of secretion in respiratory tract infections.

(4) To ensure maximum efficiency of mechanical ventilation.

The patient with a trachaeostomy cannot talk nor can he cough; also because the air he breathes goes directly into his throat, it is not filtered or moistened in his nose and will need humidifying. In addition the patient's sense of smell will be very much less sensitive than usual because air is not passing up his nose.

24

The Digestive System

The digestive system consists of a number of organs forming the alimentary or gastro-intestinal tract which extends from the mouth, where food and water enter the body, to the rectum from whence solid but lubricated waste products are excreted. The function of the system is to extract from food by chemical action the substances the body requires for growth and repair of the tissues and for the storage of energy. This is done by converting the food into compounds which can be absorbed into the blood stream which, with the lymphatic system, carry these compounds all round the body.

The Alimentary Tract

The alimentary tract is more than 9 m long (32 ft approx.) and is lined with a mucous membrane which being lubricated with mucus allows food to pass easily along. At various points chemicals enter the canal to digest the food in it.

The course of the tract is straight down from the mouth to the stomach but after the stomach it becomes very folded and descends about a median line, rises on the right side, the ascending colon, to about 12 cm (5 in) below the stomach, crosses to the left side and descends as the descending colon to the anus.

The alimentary tract is made up of six basic units:

(1) *The mouth* is the part where the food is broken up by the teeth and mixed with saliva.

(2) *The pharynx* is the cavity at the back of the mouth. Food and air pass down it but the action of swallowing closes the entrance to the larynx to prevent food from entering it. The unconscious patient may have his choking reflex damaged and can drown in his own vomit.

(3) *The oesophagus* is a muscular tube about 25 cm (10 in) long and leads to the stomach. Its muscular coat has a peristaltic action; that is to say a wave movement along the tube drives the food to the stomach.

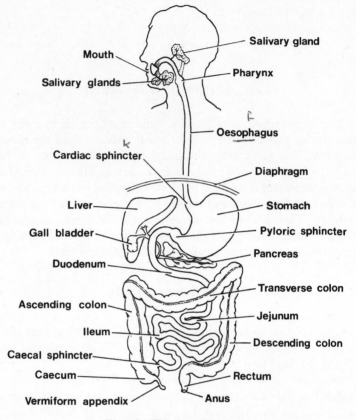

Fig. 18. The digestive tract.

(4) *The stomach* is a muscular bag high on the left side of the abdomen which receives the food. Here the food is churned up by the action of the muscular wall of the stomach and mixed with the gastric juices secreted by the lining. Gastric juice comprises principally water, hydrochloric acid and pepsinogen which is converted by the acid into pepsin and rennin. Pepsin and rennin are two enzymes which break down proteins and caseinogen. The acid also serves to kill bacteria.

(5) *The small intestine* is about 6 m (20 ft) long and is made up of duodenum, a common site of ulceration, the jejunum and the ileum. The wall of this part of the tract is arranged in folds with minute

fingerlike projections called villi which by greatly increasing the surface area enable digested food to be absorbed.

(6) *The large intestine* is the last part of the alimentary canal and here a great deal of water is absorbed and food residues prepared for evacuation. Like the small intestine it consists of three parts. The first is the caecum, a small blind pouch at whose end is the appendix 7–10 cm (3–4 in) long which in man seems to serve no purpose. The second is the colon and the last the rectum. The lower end of the rectum is guarded by a sphincter muscle 5 cm (2 in) long called the anus.

The Accessory Organs of Digestion

These are the organs which lie close to the alimentary tract and secrete digestive juices into it to act on the food as it passes by. They are the liver, gall bladder and pancreas.

The liver

The liver is the largest organ in the body and is made up of a large number of small lobes or lobules. Oxygen-rich blood enters by the hepatic artery and blood rich in nourishment, though deficient in oxygen, enters by the portal vein. Glucose is stored as glycogen here. The liver manufactures bile which helps to break down fat for digestion, though if no food is present in the stomach the bile is stored and concentrated in the gall bladder.

The gall bladder

This organ lies immediately below the liver from which it obtains bile. It is not uncommon for a stone to grow in the gall bladder giving considerable pain. Surgical removal of the gall bladder (cholecystectomy) causes little or usually no inconvenience to the patient afterwards.

The pancreas

This organ serves two purposes, the internal secretion of insulin which enables sugar to be absorbed and the external secretion of digestive juice containing amylase, lipase and trypsin.

Enzymes

An enzyme is what one might call a chemical trigger as it sets off a chemical change without being itself changed. The digestive enzymes which are secreted into the alimentary tract combine the food with water so that the food is split into simpler compounds which can be absorbed into the blood. Each enzyme has a specific role and enzyme names reflect their function, proteases acting on proteins, lipases on lipids (fats) and amylases on carbohydrates (carbohydrates contain a chemical group called an amyl radical). Digestion starts in the mouth with the enzymes in the saliva and continues in the stomach and intestines.

Enzymes are very heat sensitive and those found in the body work best at body temperature. This is why junket is made at blood temperature and why fruit and vegetables, which are going to be preserved are heated rapidly to boiling temperature, 100°C (212°F), to destroy the enzymes which would otherwise quicken their rate of decomposition.

Sphincter Muscles

The gastro-intestinal tract is a long tube open at each end; there are four places along it where the tube closes to control the rate at which the food in it moves along and to ensure that it travels in only one direction.

The four sphincters are:

(1) The cardiac sphincter, located at the entry to the stomach.
(2) The pyloric sphincter, located at the exit from the stomach.
(3) The ileocaecal sphincter, located between the ileum and colon.
(4) The anal sphincter, located at the end of the rectum.

The cardiac sphincter muscle is not very strong and though it retains food in the stomach if we remain upright it will often allow food to pass back up the oesophagus of a child who stands on his head very soon after a meal or of an older person who bends down. If the muscle becomes very weak the stomach can herniate through the diaphragm and cause constant discomfort and frequent vomiting in a condition known as hiatus hernia. This may be treated surgically or more simply by eating smaller meals and by general loss of weight. The weakness of the cardiac sphincter is not entirely an undesirable quality. If we eat something unpleasant or even poisonous we can vomit usually by reflex action but sometimes deliberately to get rid of it; a very powerful sphincter would prevent this. If the anal sphincter becomes weakened the person may suffer from faecal incontinence.

Faeces

Normal faeces are formed fairly soft and coloured brown and any variation from this should be noted. In constipation the faeces are hard and dry because they have remained too long in the colon and passage of stools is painful. An enema may be ordered to soften them and ease evacuation. The colour of faeces is an indication of good health or illness. A red colouration arises from blood which has not been digested (occult blood), whereas a black and tarry stool is evidence of the entry of blood early in the digestive tract and therefore digested; this is known as a melaena stool. Blackness alone is caused by iron or bismuth drugs and a pale clay colour shows absence of bile. A pebbly appearance in a formed stool indicates inefficient digestion arising from shortage of hydrochloric acid.

Diarrhoea, the frequent passage of fluid stools, shows that passage through the digestive tract and particularly through the large intestine (the colon) has been too rapid and water has not been extracted. In severe cases dehydration will ensue. It is particularly dangerous in a hot climate.

A child may be admitted to hospital because he has swallowed something such as a button, or the glass eye of a teddy-bear. The stools will be collected and examined to see when the foreign body has been expelled.

Worms may be seen, either round or flat, but their presence in the faeces does not mean that there are none left in the alimentary tract. Flat worms in particular usually break up leaving a head fixed to the intestinal wall, a head which will grow another body.

Faecal specimens for examination may be kept in a covered bedpan, preferably for no more than one hour and those for laboratory examination put into a sterile screw-topped specimen jar, labelled and sent to the laboratory.

Colostomy and Ileostomy

Colostomy. If there is disease or obstruction of the colon or rectum, an opening is made on the left side of the abdomen. The colon is brought to this opening, stitched into place and, if the colostomy is to be permanent, cut so that the diseased portion of the colon can be removed. The opening is known as a stoma and through it the faecal waste discharges into a plastic bag held in position by a belt. Many people have had this operation and lead normal lives, their condition being known only to the doctor and their family. The nurse plays an enormous part in helping the patient to adjust to what is at first a frightening and unwholesome situation.

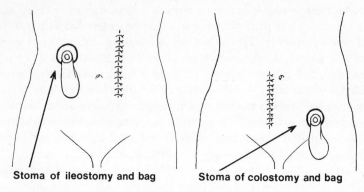

Stoma of ileostomy and bag   Stoma of colostomy and bag

Fig. 19. Positions of incision and stoma of patients with ileostomy and colostomy operations.

Ileostomy. If the entire colon and rectum are affected by disease an opening is made in the lower right abdomen, the ileum brought to the surface and a bag attached to collect the faeces.

Common Diseases and Disorders

Symptoms include nausea, abdominal pain, diarrhoea, vomiting, and constipation; none is diagnostic of disease in the digestive system though any of them repeated gives cause for concern. A further difficulty in diagnosis and treatment arises from the digestive tract's sensitivity to the emotions.

Ulcerative colitis (inflammation of the colon): stools, fluid and offensive, contain mucus and blood; treatment: bed rest, antispasmodics, blood transfusion if patient is anaemic.

Diverticulitis (multiple small pouches develop in the colon and become inflamed); treatment: bland non-residue diet with lubricating aperient; for peritonitis bed rest and antibiotics or sulphonamides.

Peptic ulcers (ulcer in the stomach or top of duodenum): acid, always present in the gastric juice, attacks the mucous membrane of some patients; treatment: bed rest and bland diet, basically milk, and administration of alkalis.

Coeliac disease (sensitivity to gluten in wheat flour causing inability to absorb fat from the small intestine): stools bulky, offensive, pale, child is thin and anaemic; treatment: gluten-free diet (see p. 19).

25

Blood and Lymph

The Blood System

Any living organism needs a system which will take nourishment to all of its parts and which removes waste products. In the higher animals this function is carried out by blood, a liquid which carries dissolved and particulate material. The liquid is plasma and the particles are blood corpuscles.

Plasma

This is a clear, pale yellow liquid, 90 per cent water which contains:

(1) Plasma proteins.
(2) Simple foodstuffs.
(3) Mineral salts.
(4) Dissolved gases, oxygen, nitrogen and carbon dioxide.
(5) Hormones.
(6) Antibodies and antitoxins.
(7) Enzymes which enable chemical reactions of metabolism to occur.
(8) Waste products of metabolism.

Blood corpuscles (cells)

These are of three types:

(1) Red blood cells: Erythrocytes.
(2) White blood cells: Leucocytes.
(3) Platelets: Thrombocytes.

The red blood cells are very small disc-shaped oxygen carriers; there are about five million in a cubic millimetre. The red colour in the cells comes from the haemoglobin which has a great affinity for oxygen. Iron is an essential constituent of haemoglobin and mildly anaemic people are often prescribed drugs containing an iron compound.

The white blood cells are very much larger, 7–8 thousand in a cubic millimetre, and their function is to combat infection.

Platelets provide a defence and repair mechanism by enabling the blood to clot. A cut will bleed and then seal itself if it is small, but when a major blood vessel is severed the flow is so rapid that the clot forming at the wound is swept away. This is why a pad is applied to staunch the flow to give time for a clot to form; severe wounds must be stitched.

Blood Transfusion and Blood Grouping

When a patient has lost a lot of blood, a blood transfusion may be the only thing to save his life. It may also be used to supplement inadequate blood formation in anaemia and leukaemia and in preparation for major surgery.

Although all blood contains the same basic constituents there are certain differences that are extremely important. If a patient receives blood that does not mix properly with his own, there can be serious, even fatal, consequences.

Some people's blood corpuscles have substances called antigens (agglutinogens) on their surface, differing according to their inherited blood group which will make them stick together in clumps if mixed with incompatible blood. The plasma of each person's blood contains antibodies which make transfused red corpuscles clump if they have the wrong antigens on their surface. It has been found that, on the basis of the presence or absence of these antigens and agglutinins, human blood falls into four groups called A, B, AB and O (no antigens) and everyone's blood belongs to one or other of these groups. When giving a blood transfusion it is vital to test both the donor's and the recipient's blood by mixing a small amount of both together to see if they are compatible.

Blood Transfusion: Donor/Recipient Compatibility

Donor	Recipient	Recipient	Donor
A	A or AB	A	A or O
B	B or AB	B	B or O
AB	AB only	AB	A, B, AB or O
O	A, AB, B or O	O	O

Rhesus factor. Another substance that may be present in the red cells is called the Rhesus factor. Those who have it (eighty-five per cent of the population) are called Rhesus positive (Rh+). Those who do not have it (fifteen per cent) are called Rhesus negative (Rh−). If Rhesus positive blood is given to a Rhesus negative person it does not appear to do immediate harm, but will stimulate the formation of antibodies, which may cause blood destruction if at a later date a further Rhesus positive transfusion is given.

If a Rhesus negative mother has a baby who inherits his father's Rhesus positive factor, the same antibodies can be made in the mother's blood which can act against the blood of a second or subsequent baby, destroying its corpuscles so that the infant will need urgent blood replacement at birth. (The mother's antibodies cross into the baby's blood stream at the placenta.) This illustrates that it is vital for all blood bottles to be checked very carefully before blood is given, both in the laboratory and in the ward. Intravenous infusions and blood transfusions are always given by the doctor but the nurse will be called upon to prepare the apparatus, look after the patient and assist the doctor.

Nursing care of a patient receiving a blood transfusion

A patient may feel apprehensive at the thought of such a procedure, and the nurse must make sure that he understands what it is all about and reassures him that it is not painful. If notice has been given of the time that the transfusion will begin, it is a good thing to encourage the patient to empty his bladder before this time. He may, if fit enough, have a wash or blanket bath and have his bed made up with clean linen. In all cases the patient must be made comfortable. During the procedure the nurse has two responsibilities. The first one is to observe the patient carefully the whole time, checking his pulse, temperature and colour. She must also assist the doctor, pouring out the lotion as he needs it and generally anticipating his wants.

After the transfusion has been set up the nurse should be given instructions about the regulation of the speed of flow of the blood and it is her duty to observe the patient frequently afterwards, so that any complication can be reported. Complications to be looked for include stopping of the flow as a result of clotting in the tube, blockage of the needle in the vein, or kinking of the tube. The patient's arm may become sore and swollen at the site of the infusion or infected if aseptic precautions are not taken.

If a second bottle of blood is to be given it is important to change the bottles before the first one is completely empty. If air is allowed to get into the patient's vein a fatal air embolus could result. There should be the same careful checking of each bottle of blood before it is given as was carried out for the first one. The nurse should again watch the patient's pulse, temperature and colour to be sure that all is well, and note any cough. All the fluid given by transfusion should be entered on a fluid chart. When the transfusion is finished the tubing is clipped, the cannula removed and the puncture covered with a sterile dressing and a firm piece of strapping until it is healed.

Mis-matched blood. The first 50–100 ml of blood are transfused very slowly and the recipient's condition watched closely. Immediate symptoms of blood of the wrong type being transfused are shivering, restlessness, nausea and vomiting, a cold and clammy skin showing cyanosis and general lumbar pain. If the infusion is not immediately stopped the pulse and respiration rates will increase and the recipient's temperature will rise to 38–40°C (100·5–104°F).

Disorders of the Blood

Anaemia is the reduced oxygen carrying capacity of the blood due to reduction in the number of red cells or the amount of haemoglobin in each red cell.

It arises from:

(1) Blood loss.
(2) Blood destruction.
(3) Lack of some factor necessary for blood formation.
(4) Some defect in bone marrow.

General signs all result from a deficient supply to the body. They are:

(1) Pallor of skin and mucous membranes.
(2) Weakness, giddiness, fainting, fatigue, loss of energy, amenorrhoea, inability to concentrate, tachycardia, palpitations, dyspnoea, heart failure, anorexia and paraesthesia.

Leukaemia is the term given to a form of cancer of the blood in which there is gross overproduction of white blood cells. This means that the proportion of red cells is reduced so severely as to cause death.

Polycythemia. In this disease there is an increase in the production of red cells. There may either be an increase of total blood volume or an increase in the number of red cells per unit of blood.

Haemophilia. In this usually hereditary disease the blood fails to clot either entirely or partially. Open wounds therefore bleed and do not seal themselves, and during an operation the clotting factor, called Factor VIII, may be injected. Blood sometimes haemorrhages into the tissues and joints causing considerable pain.

Circulation of Blood

The circulatory system consists of four distinct units whose purpose is to take the nutriments in the blood to the tissues which require them. They are described as follows:

(1) The heart which pumps the blood.
(2) The arteries which carry blood rich in oxygen to the tissues.
(3) The capillary bed, the end point of the whole process, where exchange of food and oxygen and waste products takes place.
(4) The veins which carry the blood back to the heart.

The heart

The heart is a hollow muscular organ about the size of its owner's clenched fist. It lies slightly to the left of the mid-line between the lungs and is divided into two distinct halves. Each half consists of two chambers, one of which, the atrium, receives the blood and the second, the ventricle, which discharges the blood from the heart.

The flow of blood is in the following sequence:

(1) Blood replenished with oxygen from the lungs via the four pulmonary veins enters the left atrium.
(2) The left atrium contracts driving the blood into the left ventricle.
(3) The left ventricle contracts driving the blood into the aorta and from the aorta outwards to the capillaries.
Then towards the heart:
(4) Via the two large veins, the superior vena cava and the inferior vena cava into the right atrium.

(5) The right atrium contracts driving the dark oxygen-depleted blood into the right ventricle.

(6) The right ventricle contracts driving the blood via the pulmonary trunk into the right and left pulmonary arteries and then to the lungs to be replenished with oxygen and to give up carbon dioxide and water vapour.

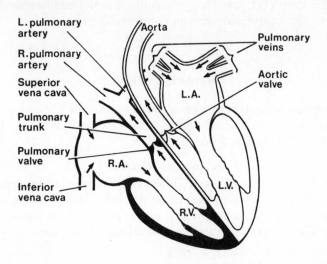

Fig. 20. Section through the heart. Arrows indicate direction of blood flow. *R.A: Right auricle. R.V: Right ventricle. L.A: Left auricle. L.V: Left ventricle.*

The heart itself, is supplied by the coronary arteries encircling it. The heart contains valves which allow blood to flow in one direction only.

The arteries

These are the thick walled vessels which carry bright red oxygenated blood out to the tissues. Note two exceptions: the left and right pulmonary arteries carry blood deficient in oxygen from the heart to the lungs.

The capillary bed

The main arteries separate into branches which repeatedly further divide until the blood flows very slowly in fine, microscopically small arterioles. Through the walls of these arterioles food, oxygen and water pass into the tissues. The arterioles join the venules via a fine network. The venules then unite to form the veins.

The veins

These are thin walled collapsible vessels through which the blood is returned to the heart. Note four exceptions: the four pulmonary veins carry blood rich in oxygen from the lungs to the heart.

Disorders of the Blood Vessels

Arteriosclerosis is a condition in which the walls of the arteries become hard, inelastic and do not stretch. As blood is forced into them by the beating heart, the pressure of the blood in the arteries rises sometimes to a dangerous level. Symptoms include headache, distorted vision and nose bleed. In the elderly, high blood pressure may cause a stroke or as it is otherwise known, a cerebrovascular accident (CVA).

Atherosclerosis occurs, usually in a vein, when a stationary blood clot, a thrombus, forms. Coronary thrombosis is the occlusion of a coronary vessel; the heart muscle is deprived of blood to an extent determined by the size of the vessel and thrombus.

Embolism is obstruction of a blood vessel by a moving obstacle, an embolus usually, a clot of blood or bubble of air or gas. Divers working in pressure units suffer from the 'bends' if they return to normal pressure at a rate which enables air absorbed in the blood stream to come out of solution as bubbles. The bends are at least painful and crippling and can easily kill.

Cerebrovascular accident (*CVA*) otherwise known as a stroke, is the sudden loss of a function such as speech or movement. It is evidence of loss of blood supply to some area of the brain.

Varicose veins are veins in which the valves no longer work efficiently to maintain the flow of blood in one direction. The veins become distended and can be seen on the legs. They tend to occur in people who stand for long periods without walking and also in pregnant women.

Haemorrhoids (piles) are varicose veins in the rectum.

Heart Disease

Heart disease may arise in any of the structures of the heart, i.e. in:

(1) The wall. The wall of the heart comprises three layers:
    (a) The pericardium, the outer double layer of serous membrane.
    (b) The myocardium, the middle layer of muscle.
    (c) The endocardium, the inner layer which includes the valves of the heart.
(2) The left side.
(3) The right side.
(4) The blood vessels to and from the heart.
(5) The coronary arteries, the left and the right which supply the heart's own muscle, the myocardium.
(6) The valves of the blood vessels and chambers.

Symptoms. According to which part of the heart is damaged or diseased, one or more of the following signs will be noticed:

(1) Dyspnoea, which is difficulty with breathing particularly during and after exertion.
(2) Pain in the chest.
(3) Palpitations, a throbbing sensation of the heart or of blood vessels in the neck.
(4) Oedema, excess fluid in the tissues.
(5) Cyanosis, blueness of the lips and skin, particularly noticeable in babies and hence the term 'blue baby'. It indicates the lack of oxygen.
(6) Haemoptysis, the coughing up of blood.
(7) Syncope, brief loss of consciousness.

None of these is on its own an indication of heart disease, cyanosis for example being seen in people with carbon monoxide gas poisoning. In addition damage in one part of the heart commonly leads to damage in another so that the patient's condition will deteriorate irreversibly unless therapy is started promptly. This will involve the use of drugs. In heart disease the morale of the patient plays an enormous part in his treatment and prognosis. The nurse must be calm and reassuring because the heart itself is very sensitive to the emotional state of the patient. If he is to be moved to another ward or hospital the cardiac patient should be told well before the time for his transfer and the move must be done quietly and without fuss.

Ischaemic heart disease

This is the commonest heat disease and the commonest single cause of death in the rich countries of the world. Ischaemic means lacking in blood and in this context refers to shortage of blood in the heart muscle, the myocardium, because the left or right pulmonary arteries are made narrower by deposits along their inner walls, athero-sclerosis. The patient may suffer attacks of severe pain in the chest extending down the left arm, a symptom called angina pectoris.

If a coronary artery becomes blocked by a clot of blood (a thrombus) the muscle fed by that artery will become necrosed. A blockage of this type is known as a coronary thrombosis.

Endocarditis

Inflammation of the endocardium, which includes the surfaces of the heart valves may be caused by a number of species of bacteria. The efficiency of the valves is impaired so that they do not close fully and thereby reduce the overall efficiency of the heart. Endocarditis usually arises from some distant focus of infection such as a bad tooth.

Pericarditis

The outer, double layer, of the heart is inflamed and excessive serum may be secreted into the area between the two layers. This will make it difficult for the heart to work to its normal capacity.

Left-sided heart failure

This refers to a state in which the blood is no longer pumped efficiently from the lungs to the arteries and capillary bed. This causes pooling of fluid and then of the blood in the lungs. Pulmonary oedema follows and leads to cardiac asthma and haemoptysis, a situation accentuated at night when the patient is lying down.

Right-sided heart failure

In this condition blood is not removed adequately from the capillary bed and veins with the result that venous pressure rises. There may initially be oedema of the ankles and feet which disappears when the patient lies down.

Drugs used in heart disease

The drugs used in heart disease are many in number but the names of a few should be remembered They may be classified according to the effects they produce as follows:

(1) Increase of heart rate. Adrenaline may be administered either by hypodermic or intravenous injection and in an emergency directly into the heart. Isoprenaline may be taken in tablet form dissolved under the tongue, or in aerosols. It also dilates the arterioles and therefore reduces blood pressure.

(2) Decrease of heart rate. Digoxin is derived from digitalis. It may be administered either by intramuscular or intravenous injection or orally. It is quick-acting and its effects last up to five days. Digitoxin is derived from another form of digitalis. It may be administered either intravenously or orally; it is slow-acting. Its effects last up to eighteen days.

(3) Maintenance of an even heart rate, i.e. beta-blocking. The nerve endings in the myocardium, called beta-receptors, are stimulated by adrenaline which is released by the adrenal glands at times of emotional or physical stress. To prevent this, drugs called beta-blocking agents are administered orally. Propranolol reduces the degree and frequency of angina pectoris but has some undesirable side-effects including dizziness and vomiting. Proctolol is similar to propranolol but has fewer side-effects. It also is given orally.

(4) Vasodilation. Glyceryl trinitrate in tablet form may be bitten and then dissolved under the tongue. It takes effect in two minutes and is effective for a quarter of an hour.

(5) Vasoconstriction. Noradrenaline is powerful but its effect is short. It is administered slowly by intravenous infusion.

(6) Hypotension, i.e. reduction of high blood pressure (hypertension). Because hypertension is so common in the rich nations an enormous number of drugs has been produced. Many are based on reserpine which is extracted from the plant Rauwolfia.

(7) Anticoagulation. Heparin administered intravenously is quickly effective for a few hours; it prevents the formation of clots.

Warfarin sodium is administered intravenously, intramuscularly or orally.

(8) Diuresis. Frusemide gives rapid diuresis taken orally.

(9) Sedation. The physician will prescribe according to the patient's particular heart condition.

(10) Antibiosis (antibiotics). In bacterial endocarditis, for example, a broad-spectrum antibiotic may be given until laboratory investi-

gation reveals the specific organism. Then an antibiotic specific to that bacterium will be prescribed.

The cardiac patient may be supplied with a wide variety of drugs to take without supervision at home and at work. The community nurse can nevertheless check that the patient is following the instructions given to him about the drugs, about his daily diet and about his general life style.

Oxygen. To increase the amount of oxygen leaving the capillaries the patient may be given oxygen by inhalation through a face mask. The mixture and duration prescribed must be carefully adhered to because the respiratory centre in the brain is stimulated by carbon dioxide. If this centre is not activated the breathing of the patient may be seriously reduced.

Haemorrhage

Bleeding can occur externally, when it is seen, or internally when it cannot be seen. It may come from an artery, a vein or a capillary. Arterial bleeding spurts out in rhythm with the heart beat and the blood looks bright red. Bleeding from a vein flows out in a continuous stream and is a darker red. Capillary bleeding oozes out from all parts of a wound.

Primary haemorrhage refers to bleeding which occurs on injury or at operation and is due to the cutting of a blood vessel. It is stopped by tying off the vessel, by direct pressure on the bleeding area, or by coagulating the blood by application of a cautery needle.

Reactionary haemorrhage is bleeding which occurs several hours after injury or surgery and happens when the blood pressure, returning to normal after being lowered by shock, forces a clot out of a vessel which it had been plugging or pushes a ligature off a blood vessel.

Secondary haemorrhage is bleeding which occurs seven to ten days after the injury or surgery and is due to the erosion of a blood vessel as a result of infection.

The nurse must, at frequent intervals, observe wounds carefully for signs of bleeding.

The Lymphatic System

Lymph is a colourless fluid derived from the blood. It seeps out from the capillaries into the spaces between the cells of the body. From the tissues it is collected into small vessels called lymph capillaries which begin in spaces between the cells and unite to form larger vessels

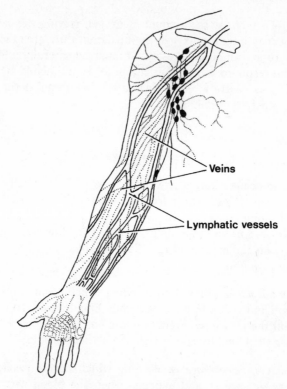

Fig. 21. The lymphatic vessels of the upper limb; lymph nodes are represented by the dark areas.

called lymph vessels. All tissues contain lymph vessels (except for nervous tissue) and eventually all drain into two large ducts which return the lymph to the blood stream at the root of the neck.

Lymph glands are found along the course of the lymphatics, some in the groin, under the arm, some in the neck and some in the pelvic and abdominal cavities, wherever a number of lymph vessels meet.

They help to filter out micro-organisms which might otherwise enter the blood stream. The lymph glands become swollen and painful as a result.

The tonsils are large lymphatic glands guarding the body against infection entering from the nose and mouth.

The spleen is the largest lymphatic gland of all. It lies in the abdominal cavity to the left of the stomach, and is about 12 cm (5 in) long. It is soft and dark in colour and holds a great deal of blood. (Damage to it is a frequent cause of internal haemorrhage in road accidents.)

The functions of the spleen are not fully understood. However they are thought to be:

(1) To produce lymphocytes for the blood stream. (Lymphocytes are involved in the production of antibodies.)

(2) To destroy red blood cells that are beginning to wear out and to break them down.

(3) To assist in fighting infection. It becomes enlarged in certain diseases where the blood is infected e.g. malaria and typhoid fever.

Tonsillitis

This is the commonest lymphatic gland disorder. Having done their work of filtering lymph and stopping unwelcome invaders like streptococci from entering the blood stream, the tonsils themselves are so full of micro-organisms that they become inflamed and painful. If pus forms the condition (a peritonsillar abscess) is called a quinsy and the abscess may have to be opened.

Hot gargles, plenty of fluids, soothing lozenges, with antibiotics and rest in bed while the temperature is high are the usual lines of treatment.

If, after several such attacks, it is decided that the tonsils are no longer able to do their work properly, the doctor may advise their removal (tonsillectomy).

26

The Urinary Systems

About three-quarters of the body's weight is made up of water which is distributed in three situations described as follows:

(1) 70 per cent inside the cells.
(2) 10 to 15 per cent as plasma and lymph.
(3) 15 to 20 per cent in intestinal spaces.

Water may pass freely between these three situations through the cell and capillary walls by diffusion and osmosis (see Chapter 20).

Water Intake and Output

A healthy person takes in approximately 2·5 l (4 pt) of water every day and excretes the same amount by natural process. 1·5 l (2·5 pt) of the daily intake is in the form of drinks such as water, tea, coffee, beer and soup and a little more than one litre is taken in the food we eat. The equalization of intake and output is known as water balance. Excretion of water is by four routes as outlined below:

(1) 1500 ml per day is excreted from the kidneys as urine.
(2) 600 ml per day is excreted from the skin as sweat.
(3) 100 ml per day is excreted from the anus in the faeces.
(4) 400 ml per day is excreted from the lungs as water vapour.

The output of urine is greater in cold weather because sweating is reduced. Conversely in a hot climate sweating is profuse and urine production is limited. Whatever the climate the urinary system plays a dominant part in maintaining water balance. This vital role will be appreciated even more when the other functions of the kidneys are understood.

The Functions of the Kidneys

The main function of the kidneys is to adjust the composition of the blood which they do by removing from it unwanted substances which include:

(1) The end products of protein metabolism, urea, uric acid, creatinine.

(2) Salts.

(3) Pigments which are derived from red cell breakdown.

The kidneys also control the amount of water remaining in the body and the acidity of the blood.

Constituents of the Urinary Systems

The kidneys

These are dark red, bean-shaped organs weighing about 130 g (5 oz), 10 cm (4 in) long, 6 cm (2·5 in) wide and 4 cm (1·5 in) thick. They lie embedded in a protective layer of fat on either side of the

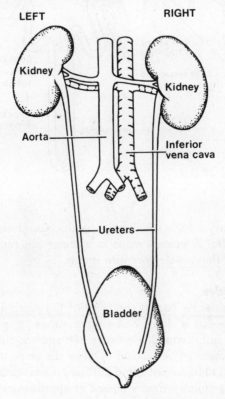

Fig. 22. The urinary system.

vertebral column and level with the lower ribs. Each kidney is encased in a capsule of fibrous tissue and lies outside the peritoneum. Its three main parts are the cortex, the medulla and the pelvis. The pelvis conveys the urine to the ureters.

The ureters

The ureters drain the urine from the kidneys to the urinary bladder. They are about 25 cm (10 in) long and their walls contain

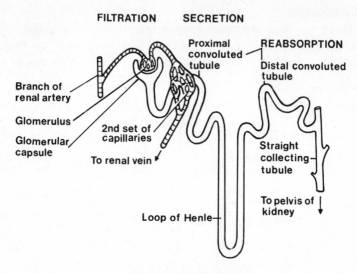

Fig. 23. A nephron.

some involuntary muscle which by peristaltic action directs the urine into the bladder. A urinary stone in a ureter can cause severe pain (renal colic) if the muscle goes into spasm.

Urinary bladder

This is a muscular bag in the front of the pelvis into which the urine flows; its exit is closed by a ring of muscle, a sphincter. When the bladder is full it contains between 180 and 500 ml (0·25 to 1 pt) and the sphincter can be relaxed to allow the urine to escape down the urethra and to be passed out of the body; this is called micturition. During waking hours urine is passed at approximately four-hourly intervals.

The nephron

The working unit of the kidney is the nephron which is so small as to be visible only under the microscope; each kidney contains approximately a million. Each nephron is a very fine tube, or tubule, which leads from the renal artery (they are not directly connected) to the pelvis of the kidney where urine discharges into the ureters.

The end of the tubule in contact with the renal artery is cup-shaped; into this cup, called the glomerular capsule, enters a fine tuft of renal artery capillaries called a glomerulus. The kidney is very close to the aorta with the result that the blood pressure in the glomerulus is very high.

Urine

The production of urine

Urine is produced by:

(1) Filtration; (2) Reabsorption; (3) Secretion.

The blood entering the kidneys by the renal arteries carries the soluble waste products from the body; it also carries, as does all blood, water, salts and glucose which the body needs. Filtration of enormous volumes (150 l per day) occurs between the capillary tuft and the glomerular capsule though, because most of the filtered liquid is reabsorbed into the blood stream from the distal tubules, only 1·5 l of urine is produced.

Selective reabsorption of salts and glucose takes place at the second set of capillaries; it is here that secretion also occurs, potassium for example leaving the blood system to enter the walls of the tubules and thence by the tubules going to the bladder.

Composition and characteristics of urine

The urine of a healthy person is composed of water in which are dissolved soluble waste products of metabolism, namely inorganic mineral salts and organic compounds in the proportions:

Water: 96 per cent.
Urea: 2 per cent.
Uric acid and salts: 2 per cent.

Urine is normally sterile.

Urine must be examined as a matter of course and the nurse must look briefly at any specimen passed into a bottle or bedpan. This does not mean that tests have to be done on every specimen; it is sufficient to note the colour, clarity and quantity and smell.

Colour. Normal urine is pale yellow to amber. The colour is a rough indication of the amount of liquid drunk, the paler the colour, the greater the quantity.

A dark brown colour sometimes seen with a greenish tinge indicates the presence of bile pigments; it is seen in a jaundiced patient. A smoky appearance indicates that a little blood may be present, whilst a red colour indicates the presence of copious blood. A check should be made on the drug regimen which might be the cause of this colour. A green colour may also be due to the administration of some drugs.

Clarity. Urine of whatever tint of yellow should be completely clear in a healthy person. Cloudiness may be caused by disease or by precipitation of salts when the urine is allowed to stand.

Quantity. The amount passed at any one time need not be accurately measured unless a check is being kept on the patient's fluid balance. It is important that a bedridden person drinks enough to maintain production of urine. If a nurse notices that someone is drinking unusually large amounts or passing very large or small amounts she must enter the facts in the patient's notes and tell the doctor.

Tests

Specific gravity, which means the heaviness of the urine compared to water which is given the value 1·000, is measured with a special float called a urinometer. The urinometer floats in the urine and where the surface of the urine touches the scale on the urinometer the specific gravity, s.g. is read off. Its value is normally between 1·015 and 1·025.

Acidity. If a drop of urine is put onto a piece of blue litmus paper the paper will turn red if the urine is acid.

Odour. Urine has an odour recognizably its own. A fishy odour may be caused by infection and a smell of acetone sometimes arises in diabetes.

There are a number of proprietary kits for testing urine for albumen, sugar, blood, acetone or bile pigment.

Collection of specimen

The tests which may be carried out by the nurse in the ward or sluice, determine the presence or absence of chemicals and blood. They do not indicate either infection in the urinary tract or elsewhere. Diagnosis of a urinary tract infection can be confirmed only by bacteriological examination of urine in the laboratory. The urine sent for examination must be free of all contamination by micro-organisms on the perineum (near the urethra) or a false diagnosis may be made.

Urine is a good medium for the growth and multiplication of micro-organisms and it must for this reason be collected at a time when it can quickly be sent to the laboratory. If delay cannot be avoided the specimen is placed in a refrigerator at once.

Midstream specimen. The following articles are taken to the patient's bedside:

Small sterile bowl holding tap water.
Packet of sterile swabs for cleaning around the urethra.
Sterile jar with screw-top.
Sterile receiver for collecting urine.
Clean receiver and paper bag for swabs.

The patient, whenever possible, carries out the procedure though the nurse must make sure that her instructions are followed. She gives the female patient a clean bedpan and a man a clean urine bottle.

In women the vulva is parted and the urethral area cleaned with a moist sterile swab, the direction being from the front backwards; the urethral orifice is dried with another sterile swab. The patient starts to pass urine into the bedpan and uses the sterile receiver to catch 10 to 12 ml a few seconds after the stream has started. The nurse transfers this specimen to the sterile screwtop jar which is labelled for identification. Note: label the jar not the lid. If a midstream specimen cannot be obtained the sterile receiver is placed in the bedpan, its contents are as before put into the sterile jar. The specimen is labelled *'clean urine specimen'*.

In men the glans penis is washed with a sterile swab dipped in tap water and dried with another sterile swab. The procedure is most easily carried out if the patient can stand over a lavatory bowl and catch a midstream specimen in the sterile receiver which the nurse later transfers to the screwtop jar.

Catheterization

There is always the possibility, when catheterizing a patient, of introducing infection and of causing physical damage to the urethra. A catheter is therefore introduced only when essential. Many patients will be embarrassed and some frightened at the prospect of catheterization. The bed is screened and the procedure is carefully explained.

Catheter toilet

This is used for patients who have an indwelling catheter and is a clean but not sterile procedure. If possible each patient has his own tray holding:

A clean gallipot.
A pack of gauze swabs.
Paper bag for used swabs.
0·5 per cent aqueous Hibitane.
Patient's own towel, soap and back flannel.

After washing the patient's groins the nurse washes her own hands. External genitalia, urethral orifice and catheter are cleaned with swabs dipped into the Hibitane and used once only. This is done not less than three times a day. Men can usually do this themselves. Urine bags are best changed during the day so that patients have undisturbed nights. Specimens can be obtained at the same time.

Some Disorders of the Urinary System

Abnormal micturition

Retention may be caused by an unaccustomed position in bed necessary after an operation. It may be prevented by making the patient pass urine while in bed before the operation. A warm drink, application of heat over the lower abdomen and the sound of running water may stimulate the patient to pass urine. There may be obstruction in the urethra. A catheter should be passed only when all other methods have failed because of the risk of introducing infection.

Retention with overflow is due to obstruction of the neck of the bladder, urine being passed only when the pressure of urine in the bladder is great enough to overcome the obstruction. It may also arise from loss of elasticity in the sphincter muscle caused by prolonged retention and stretching of the bladder wall in retention of urine. The bladder is full but urine dribbles constantly.

Incontinence. The bladder fails to retain urine when muscular weakness occurs, commonly in elderly or bedridden people. It also occurs in paraplegia, when the lower part of the body is paralysed, or following a stroke.

Increased frequency. Micturition takes place more often than normal during waking hours. It may be caused by irritation, infection, disease, pressure or anxiety.

Suppression occurs if the kidneys fail to manufacture urine or when the ureters are blocked. The condition must be reported immediately.

Enuresis or bedwetting is the incontinence of childhood and may arise from faulty training, anxiety or to being cold in bed. It often starts after the birth of a baby brother or sister. Scolding and punishment are likely to extend rather than cure enuresis.

Acute nephritis

This is an acute inflammatory condition arising from the kidney's allergic reaction to the toxins of a streptococcal infection. The patient may have had a sore throat for two or three weeks and now has a puffiness around the eyes and typically an increase in weight caused by oedema. Urinary output will be considerably decreased, oliguria, and the urine will appear dark and smoky. The patient may feel generally ill and his temperature will be raised. He may experience rigor and children may even have convulsions.

Investigations will include tests for blood in the urine, haematuria, and for cell casts. These casts are peculiar to an inflammatory condition of the tubules whose linings flake off and are passed in the urine. In addition the physician will carry out a full investigation to detect any hidden infection arising in the teeth, tonsils or sinuses.

Treatment consists of measures to rest both the patient and his kidneys. Therefore he must be in bed and his fluid intake limited to 1·5 l (2 pt) or less each day. The diet forms a very important part of treatment and is designed to lessen the risk of uraemia. Protein is restricted to 20–30 g (1 oz) per day but carbohydrates will prevent the breakdown of body protein and will provide adequate calorie intake. No salt is allowed and the fluid will have glucose added to it. When diuresis increases fluid intake is also increased by the same amount and under the strictest supervision the diet can now include vegetables, milk, eggs or fish, but only when improvement is complete can meat be included. Nursing care will be as for any feverish patient and special attention must be paid to turning the patient who will be oedematous and who will need a daily blanket bath because he will perspire a great deal.

Nephrotic syndrome

In this condition the urine is loaded with albumen and the oedema which occurs only on the face in acute nephritis, extends over the whole body and is seen clearly in the legs, trunk and genitalia. The face is pale and heavy and the eyelids so heavy that the patient may not be able to keep his eyes open. There is no problem with passing waste material in the urine and the patient can be given a diet rich in protein, though as with acute nephritis salt intake must be low. Complete recovery is unlikely and patients are encouraged to become active as soon as their condition allows.

Nursing care is the same as for acute nephritis with added emphasis on avoidance of pressure sores.

Chronic renal failure

Uraemia is the term used to describe the clinical syndrome which is the result of renal failure. This is a somewhat misleading word because though urea is the chief waste substance there are others. The kidneys can no longer remove the toxic products of metabolism which therefore accumulate in the body. The outcome of kidney failure is fatal unless a kidney from another person can be transplanted. The blood can be artificially cleared of its toxins by a process of dialysis in an artificial kidney machine though it must be realized that dialysis is not a cure. Every system of the body is affected, the patient becomes drowsy and even comatose, his tongue and skin are dry and his breath smells of urine, blood pressure rises and the blood itself becomes anaemic.

Urinary tract infection

Cystitis, inflammation of the bladder, and pyelonephritis, inflammation of the pelvis of the kidney must be treated immediately. A broad-spectrum antibiotic is usually used until culture in the laboratory reveals the causative organism when an antibiotic specific to that organism is prescribed. The patient is nursed in bed and must be prompted to drink large quantities of alkaline fluids.

27

The Reproductive Systems

The human race is the most highly developed intellectual species on Earth. Nevertheless it possesses the two strongest instincts common to all animal life, namely self-preservation and continuation of the species. Man has throughout history devoted a great deal of thought and energy to the study and gratification of his sexual instinct and early religions placed great emphasis on fertility as indeed some do today.

Conception

Sexual intercourse takes place when the male penis enters the female vagina and ejaculates sperm. If only one of these two hundred million sperm reaches and penetrates her ovum the woman becomes pregnant. The haploid sperm unites with the haploid ovum to form one diploid cell. This bald description takes no account of the sense of joy and tenderness that two people in love feel for each other. The natural outcome is the birth of a baby and it is the human baby's total reliance on its mother that dictates the social structure of civilized and primitive society.

Gynaecology

At one time the gynaecologist concerned himself with the illnesses of women in so far as these illnesses were exclusive to women, i.e. disorders of the uterus. Nowadays a modern gynaecologist considers the woman totally and relates her sickness to all systems, not merely to her reproductive function. He must understand the mental stresses to which women are exposed in professional and in family life and he will be concerned with infertility and family planning, with childbirth and with cancer.

Obstetrics is the branch of medicine dealing with birth though it is often understood to be included in gynaecology.

Paediatrics is concerned with the medical and surgical treatment of infants and children.

Midwifery is the specialized branch of nursing which deals with care of the pregnant woman, delivery of her baby and the immediate aftercare of both.

The nurse in a women's surgical or medical ward will have to know about gynaecological illness in addition to other aspects of medicine. Her patients will even more than usual appreciate privacy and kindness in what are often embarrassing conditions.

Gynaecological procedures

Vaginal douche is a cleansing procedure sometimes used preoperatively for patients having repair operations and for those with a vaginal discharge. It is also used when a patient has had radium removed. The cleansing solution is mild, for example normal saline, and the method is initially the same as for catheterization, the labia being cleaned with antiseptic lotion before the rubber or glass irrigation nozzle is inserted into the vagina. 2 l of solution (about 3 pt), are required.

Removal of radium. Radium is a radioactive metal which is often used in the treatment of gynaecological cancers. The surgeon decides on the length of time for the radium to remain in position and it is therefore removed at the time specified by him. Each applicator is removed, rinsed in disinfectant and placed in the radiation-proof box which is taken immediately to the safe designed for it.

Cervical smear. To detect the earliest stage of cancer of the cervix the doctor takes a specimen of the surface cells for later examination under a microscope. The painless procedure is carried out in the doctor's surgery or at home, or for in-patients in the ward.

Gynaecological operations

Dilatation and curettage. The patient is usually examined under a general anaesthetic in the theatre. The cervix is dilated and the lining of the endometrium scraped. The purpose is usually to clean up after a heavy period, an incomplete spontaneous abortion, or for diagnosis.

Hysterectomy is the operation for total removal of the uterus and while women who have had children may accept their improved condition happily, younger women will suffer acute distress because in addition to their inability to have children they often believe that their femininity will decline.

Hysterectomy with salpingo-oophorectomy. In this operation the ovarian tubes and ovaries are removed as well as the uterus. The physician may institute hormone therapy to compensate for the loss of hormones from the ovaries.

Prolapse. If the muscular floor of the pelvic cavity becomes weak abdominal organs may herniate into the vaginal wall as follows:

(1) Cystocele: The urinary bladder herniates into the anterior wall of the vagina.

(2) Rectocele: The rectum herniates into the posterior wall.

(3) Prolapse of the uterus into the vagina.

Surgical correction will be needed for each of these forms of prolapse.

Caesarean section. If a mother, or her baby, is suffering or likely to suffer excessively from a prolonged labour the obstetrician may decide to deliver the fetus through an incision made in the wall of the abdomen and in the uterus; Julius Caesar is said to have been born in this way.

The Male Reproductive System

The male reproductive system consists of the following:

The testes, a pair of glandular organs which manufacture spermatozoa (male sex cells) and the seminal fluid in which they swim. At the upper end of each testis is an epididymis in which the sperm are stored. The testes are contained in the scrotum.

The vas deferens, a duct connecting the epididymis to the urethra. It is the route by which sperm enter the urethra.

The seminal vesicles which store a sticky fluid which forms part of the semen. They lie posteriorly to the urinary bladder on either side of the prostate gland.

The prostate gland is a muscular gland which lies at the base of the bladder and surrounds the urethra; it is about 2·5 cm (1 in) across and in old age may constrict the urethra so that surgery is needed; this is commonly known as 'old man's disease'.

The penis is a spongy vascular tissue which when stimulated sexually becomes rigid. This is not a muscular mechanism but is the result of the veins draining the penis being constricted when the man is sexually aroused. The penile urethra carries both urine and semen, though there is a mechanism to prevent the passage of urine when the penis is erect.

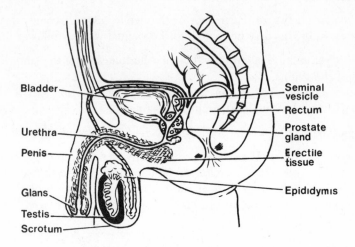

Fig. 24. Section through the male pelvis.

The Female Reproductive System

The external reproductive organs

The external genital organs of the female together comprise the vulva. They are described as follows:

The mons veneris consists of a pad of fat situated in front of the symphysis pubis, the joint where the two halves of the pelvis meet at the front. During puberty it becomes covered with hair.

The labia majora are two rounded lip-like folds of skin which extend backwards from the mons in a curve and unite in the perineum in front of the anus. Each labia contains a Bartholin's gland which secretes mucus.

The labia minora are two folds of skin lying within the labia majora. All the labia enclose a triangular area called the vestibule within which are found the openings of the urethra and vagina. In front the labia meet to form a hood-like structure called the prepuce which surrounds and protects the clitoris.

The clitoris is a small sensitive organ containing erectile tissue. It becomes firm and rigid when congested with blood which occurs during the stimulation of sexual intercourse.

The hymen is a membrane which almost completely covers the entrance to the vagina. There is a perforation in the centre which allows the menstrual discharge to escape.

The perineum is the muscle which lies between the anus and the vagina; it is quite commonly injured in a mother having her first baby.

The internal reproductive organs

The internal reproductive organs consist of the left and right ovaries, the Fallopian tubes (one from each ovary), the uterus and the vagina.

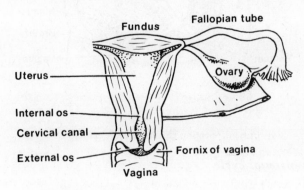

Fig. 25. The female reproductive organs.

The two ovaries are small oval glands in the pelvic cavity; each lies immediately below its Fallopian tube which forms an arch over it. Every month after puberty one ovum is released from one of the two ovaries and is carried along the Fallopian tube to the uterus to be finally discharged through the vagina with a certain amount of blood from the wall of the uterus. This process is called menstruation.

The baby girl is born with all her ova. They are not formed at puberty but develop then and are discharged at regular monthly intervals unless one is fertilized by a sperm cell.

The uterus consists of three layers. The outer one is serous peritoneum and the middle layer is involuntary muscle whose fibres run in different directions to form a crisscross network which gives very strong contractions during labour to expel the fetus through the vagina. The inner layer, the endometrium, undergoes changes during the twenty-eight day menstrual cycle to prepare to receive a fertilized ovum. If the ovum is not fertilized the lining of the uterus is shed and menstruation occurs. The discharge consists of blood, mucus, and epithelial cells and normally amounts to between 100 to 200 g (3 to 7 oz).

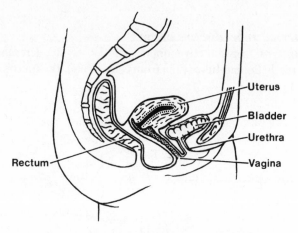

Fig. 26. Section through the female pelvis.

The menstrual cycle

The endometrium undergoes a cycle of change each month in preparation for a fertile ovum during which its walls become progressively thicker and engorged with blood until the congested blood vessels rupture and blood escapes into the uterine cavity. The bleeding continues for up to six days though this blood does not clot and therefore can flow away.

The four phases of the cycle are as follows:

(1) the premenstrual phase (initiated by ovulation) of fourteen days before the discharge is evacuated. This is the time during which the endometrium becomes thicker.

(2) menstruation which is the time of discharge.

(3) the repair stage lasting about a week.

(4) the resting phase before the next premenstrual phase.

The menstrual cycle usually follows a regular pattern but it is perfectly normal for it to be upset by happiness as much as by shock. The newly married woman often believes she has conceived when her period is a few days late.

Amenorrhoea means absence of menstruation and may be primary or secondary. Primary amenorrhoea means that menstruation has never occurred, for instance in the congenital absence of ovaries or uterus. It also arises from pituitary malfunction or as the result of serious illness such as tuberculosis.

Secondary amenorrhoea means that menstruation has occurred but has now ceased. It commonly arises as a result of mental disturbance, severe illness or hormonal disorder. It is seen in patients suffering from anorexia nervosa.

Dysmenorrhoea refers to painful periods and may be primary or secondary. Primary dysmenorrhoea is that in which after the first few periods a griping colicky pain is felt. However this usually resolves and is very unusual in women who have had a baby. Young women who have had little or no education in menstruation and who are frightened by their first periods are often cured by a full and careful explanation of what is happening to them. The patient may be prescribed a mild analgesic such as paracetamol and told to take care to avoid constipation and to take exercise. Secondary dysmenorrhoea occurs in women of between thirty and forty years of age; it is usually caused by a pathological condition and the patient should visit her doctor.

Menorrhagia. In this condition the patient has heavy and prolonged periods. The cause may be anaemia, a hormone imbalance, or may arise from polyps or fibroids. The severity may be assessed by ascertaining the number of pads or tampons used and by asking what has been the effect on social life. A cure must be made because the amount of blood lost can be considerable.

Intermenstrual bleeding may be due to carcinoma of the cervix or to hormonal changes particularly at the menopause.

Venereal diseases

These are diseases which are sexually transmitted, the two commonest being syphilis and gonorrhoea; the incidence of both has increased enormously and continues to rise so that in England and

Wales there are as many as fifty thousand new cases of gonorrhoea every year and worldwide, sixty million.

A mother can transmit syphilis to her unborn baby, and the mother with gonorrhoea may infect her baby's eyes at birth by direct contact with her genital tract, and give rise to a condition called ophthalmia neonatorum. Treatment is usually in a special clinic of a hospital where the nurse's role as counsellor and friend is as valuable as her technical skill because the social disgrace associated with venereal diseases gives many patients a deep sense of shame. To preserve confidentiality patients are usually given a number and their name is never used.

Abortion

Abortion is the termination of a pregnancy before the twenty-eighth week; it may occur without medical intervention or be performed deliberately. Threatened abortion means that the patient is experiencing vaginal bleeding and will have to rest in bed, often in hospital in order to save the pregnancy. Complete abortion indicates that all the products of conception have been expelled, whereas in inevitable abortion measures must be started to complete an abortion in which some material remains in the uterus or vaginal tract. Therapeutic abortion is an abortion carried out for medical or psychiatric reasons for the sake of the mother's well-being or because the fetus is known to be abnormal or at least very likely to be born abnormal. Habitual abortion is when a woman has aborted three or more times. Criminal abortion is one carried out by an unskilled person, that is to say by someone who is not a doctor; it is illegal.

28

The Skin

The skin is the outer covering of the body and consists of two layers. The surface layer is called the epidermis and under this lies the dermis. The epidermis varies in thickness and flexibility in different parts of the body, according to the amount of wear and tear to which it is subjected, the thickest being on the soles of the feet and the palms of the hands, and the most flexible being on the face. (Note the changes in smiling and frowning.) The epidermis consists of a number of layers of growing epithelium whose cells become flattened and

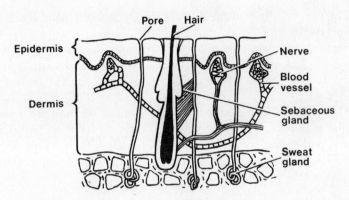

Fig. 27. Section through the skin.

are rubbed off and replaced by new ones from below. It is an example of compound or stratified epithelium. It has no blood vessels, nerves or glands and its lower layers of cells are nourished by lymph. The layer next to the dermis contains special pigment cells to protect the delicate tissues below from the sun's rays. This pigment, melanin, is slightly more in abundance in people with dark skin than in those with a lighter one.

The epidermis is thrown into ridges by projections arising from the dermis. These ridges are particularly marked on the pads of the fingers and form a pattern different in every individual, which are called fingerprints. Some maternity units record the fingerprints of all babies at birth as an additional means of identification and as a means of diagnosing some congenital abnormalities e.g. mongolism.

The dermis lies below the epidermis and is well supplied with blood and lymphatic vessels, sweat and sebaceous glands, hair follicles and nerve endings.

The glands which secrete sweat are coiled tubes whose ducts pass through the epidermis to open as pores on the surface of the skin all over the body. They are most abundant in the axillae, palms of the hands, soles of the feet and forehead. On the palms of each hand alone there are at least three thousand five hundred. The sweat which they secrete is a colourless fluid containing ninety-nine per cent water with salts, especially sodium chloride and waste products. The sebaceous glands open into the hair follicles. They secrete a fatty substance called sebum which keeps the hair glossy and the skin smooth.

The nerve endings of the skin are mainly sensory (pain, touch and temperature).

Between the dermis and deeper structures there is a layer of fat called the subcutaneous fat. This gives roundness and softness to the body. It also provides heat insulation and protects the body from injury.

The nails and hair are the appendages of the skin and are made of similar materials. The nails are modifications of the epidermis and correspond to the hoofs and claws of animals. The hairs develop in hair follicles in the skin. Their colour depends on the pigment melanin in the cells which produce them.

The areas of the trunk

It is often necessary to explain where a patient feels pain or what area of skin is to be shaved in preparation for an operation. Figure 28 shows the names given to the nine areas; these names refer to the areas and not to any organ or structures.

The functions of the skin

(1) To protect from invasion by micro-organisms and from injury.

(2) To prevent the loss of lymph and plasma.

(3) To regulate the temperature by the evaporation of sweat which takes the heat from the body and by radiation of heat.

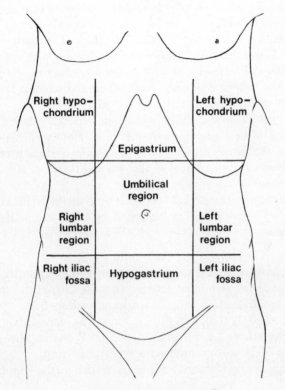

Fig. 28. Regions of the trunk.

(4) To excrete some waste matter in the sweat.

(5) To give the sensation of touch, heat, cold and pain, so making the individual aware of what is around him.

(6) To produce vitamin D, when the ultraviolet rays in sunlight fall on a fatty substance called ergosterol in the skin.

(7) To secrete sebum.

(8) To absorb small amounts of some oily substances.

Heat regulation of the body

Man is a warm-blooded creature and his normal temperature does not vary with his surroundings but remains at a constant level between 36·1 and 37·2°C (97 and 99°F) being a little lower in the morning. People who live in Iceland have the same internal temperature as those who live at the equator but when a man is ill his temperature will vary from normal.

In health the skin is firm, elastic, supple and smooth with few blemishes. These qualities deteriorate with age and with exposure to sun and wind. The colour of skin varies according to whether the patient is hot, when it becomes flushed, or cold when it takes on a blueish tint and in fright it becomes very pale.

In temperate and cold climates clothing, especially dark clothing, prevents loss of heat generated by the body. However, in a hot and dry climate, the Sahara desert for instance, white clothing protects the Bedouin from the radiant heat of the sun and therefore serves a different purpose.

The body temperature is kept constant by a careful balance between heat gain and heat loss and is controlled by a heat-regulating centre in the brain.

Heat gain. The body gains heat in three ways:

(1) By converting food to produce energy. The quantity of heat made depends on glandular activity and the amount of muscular exercise taken. In exercise muscles work and produce heat.

When the body is cold, heat production can be increased by muscular twitching otherwise known as shivering. When it takes place in the muscles of the jaw it results in the teeth 'chattering'.

(2) By absorbing from external sources such as the sun, fires and radiators.

(3) A small amount of heat can be obtained by eating and drinking hot foods.

Heat loss. Heat may be lost from the body in several ways:

(1) By the secretion and evaporation of sweat. Heat loss depends on the evaporation of sweat and this is controlled by the amount of blood passing through the vessels surrounding the sweat glands in the dermis. When the temperature of the body rises the blood vessels dilate, the skin becomes warm and pink and more sweat is made. Heat is taken from the body when sweat evaporates.

(2) By conduction, radiation and convection to the air and clothing round the body. This is noticeable after leaving a warm bed in the morning. Heat loss can be helped in hot weather and minimized in cold by wearing clothes. According to the material, colour and style these will either keep heat in or let it out. The hair, fur and feathers of animals and birds act in the same way.

(3) Heat is also lost from the body in expired air and in excreta.

Heat stroke

If the humidity or heat of the atmosphere prevents heat loss by evaporation or radiation heat stroke can occur, which can, if untreated, result in death as the temperature of the body becomes too high for metabolic processes to take place.

Fever

Fever (pyrexia) during infection is a defence on the part of the body because the high temperature makes conditions in the blood and tissues unfavourable for the growth of infecting organisms.

Routine General Care of the Skin

Personal care of the skin

It is most important that a nurse should set a good example to patients by the condition of her own skin to which regular care must be given. It can easily be affected by wind, cold and sun. Conditions such as constipation, digestive disorders and dietary indiscretions affect the skin in the form of spots, pimples, boils, sallowness and pallor.

As one of the main functions of the skin is to help regulate the temperature of the body, it should be kept clean by washing. This will keep the skin clear of the accumulations which, if left, can clog the pores and cause soreness and irritation. Nurses should remember that their hair, faces and hands will be continually on show, so great care must be taken of them. All make-up should be removed every night with a reliable cleansing cream before going to bed and skin food applied, alternatively a bland soap may be used.

It is often forgotten that hands are on show as much as the face. Certain jobs that a nurse will be required to do will necessitate the wearing of gloves for protection, but many nursing procedures are so delicate that gloves are a handicap. Nurses must also wash their hands before and after carrying out each procedure to avoid the risk of spreading infection from one patient to another. This constant washing increases the tendency to sore and chapped hands which can be relieved by the use of hand cream, so washing should be done with care with soap and warm water, the nails being cleaned with a soft bristle brush to avoid breaking the skin. Nails should be well cared for and always clean. A nurse should always wear her hair clean and in a style suitable for wearing with uniform and hair should not touch the collar.

Nurses, men as well as women will appreciate the cleansing and relaxing value of a daily bath. The application of an antiperspirant particularly to the armpits, helps keep the nurse fresh and free from odours. Now that many men are entering the nursing profession many points already mentioned will also be applicable to them. Bathing, the use of deodorants, care of the hands and hair applies equally to them. Shaving of the beard should be carried out daily, or more often if necessary.

If a nurse remembers all these points she (or he) will create an atmosphere of confidence for the many patients who pass through her hands, just by looking wholesome and healthy.

Care of the patient's skin

In her work of caring for the sick a nurse should attend to the toilet and every detail affecting the patient's well-being, in such a way as to spare him any embarrassment.

A patient should be washed twice a day and, owing to the great risk of infection being carried to the mouth and spreading through the body, the hands should always be washed after the patient has used a bedpan or been to the lavatory. If possible a bath should be given daily, but never less than once a week. It should however be remembered that the skin of the elderly has lost much of its elasticity and has a tendency to be dry, so too much washing will increase the dryness. When the patient is not given a bath his groins and buttocks must be washed at least twice a day. The temperature of the water for a tepid bath is about 32°C (90°F) cooling to about 27°C (80°F) and of a hot bath it is about 40°C (104°F). The nurse must always prepare the water for a patient's bath and test it with a bath thermometer and see that everything is in readiness; soap, towels and clean clothing. The patient may also like to go to the lavatory first. The windows must be closed and though the patient may be left alone in the bath, the door must not be locked and the nurse must be within call. A screen can be put round the bath to ensure privacy and a bell should be within reach. A cupful of common salt in the bath water guards against cross-infection between patients. After bathing she should see that the patient's body is clean, look at the finger and toenails and cut them if necessary. Abnormalities such as bruises, spots, cuts and deformities must be noted and reported at once to the sister in charge of the ward.

The bath is scrubbed out when it has been used and disinfected with the disinfectant in general use at the hospital and the bottle put away in a safe place afterwards. The windows should be opened and the bathroom left clean and tidy and ready for use by the next patient.

Bathing a patient in bed

A patient whose temperature is higher than 37·2°C (99°F) or who is too ill to go to the bathroom is bathed in bed. Two nurses will be needed if the patient is very ill or unable to move.

Individual bath blankets should be used for each patient and kept in his locker. Where it is not possible to supply individual bath blankets it is better to use the top blanket from the patient's own bed and a large towel underneath him. On no account should the same blanket be used for more than one patient for this is another way in which infection may be quickly spread around the ward.

Procedure. To give a blanket bath, the procedure is as follows:

(1) The patient is protected from draughts by closing nearby windows and the curtains are drawn round the bed.

(2) Everything that is likely to be used is prepared beforehand and the temperature of the room is checked to see that it is warm enough.

(3) The patient is offered a bedpan.

(4) The patient's clothes are put to warm.

(5) The upper bedclothes are removed and the patient covered with a warm blanket.

(6) The second bath blanket is rolled underneath him.

(7) His gown or pyjamas are removed gently and his face and neck are washed and dried thoroughly, then his arms and hands, keeping the rest of his body covered. His chest, abdomen, legs and feet are then dealt with, care being taken to wash and dry carefully between his toes.

(8) If possible the patient should be allowed to dip his hands and feet in the bowl of water. This will give great pleasure to him.

(9) The nurse must pay particular attention to the axillae, to the folds of skin under the breasts and to the umbilicus. These parts can quickly become dirty if not cared for. If the patient is able to do so, he

is allowed, under cover of the blanket, to wash his groin and genital organs. If he is helpless the nurse should do it for him, carefully and thoroughly.

(10) The water is then changed, the patient rolled over and his back and buttocks washed. It is important to keep the water really hot all the time. Only the part that is actually being washed should be uncovered. The patient must always be dried thoroughly; this will have a relaxing effect on him.

(11) All pressure areas must be examined and treated as necessary in the course of the bathing. Nails should be trimmed carefully, cutting off only a little at a time, to take the shape of his fingertips and cutting the toenails straight across to prevent the development of ingrowing toenails.

(12) At the end of the bath, the bath blanket should be rolled out, the patient dressed in his clean gown or pyjamas and his upper bed-clothes replaced. His mouth and hair should then be attended to. A hot drink is given him if he wants one, then everything is cleared away leaving him tidy and comfortable and ensuring that he has everything that he needs, including his bell.

Care of the patient's hair

The hair of all patients whose condition permits should be washed regularly if they have to stay in hospital for a long time. This has a good, uplifting effect on the patient, giving him a feeling of well-being. It may be possible for a trained hairdresser to visit the wards and do this with the help of a nurse.

The patient should be arranged in the position which distresses him the least, for instance, a patient with difficult breathing (dyspnoea) must never be made to lie on his back. The patient's shoulders should be protected with a blanket and a waterproof cape and some cotton wool lightly placed in his ears to prevent water getting in. He is also given a face towel to protect his eyes. A space is arranged for the bowl to be placed under the patient's head to facilitate rinsing. After the shampoo and rinse, the patient's hair is brushed and combed gently.

The care of the pressure areas

Patients who require special care. Special attention should be paid to the pressure areas of all bedridden patients, especially those suffering from:

(1) Incontinence, because the skin is often wet.

(2) Paralysis, when the patient cannot move from the position in which he is lying.

(3) Oedema, when the patient is not only extra heavy, but the skin is unhealthy from lack of natural circulation.

(4) Loss of weight, when the bones are just under the skin.

(5) Overweight, when pressure is unusually great.

Other patients who need special care are:

(6) Elderly patients whose tissues tend to have less vitality.

(7) Those wearing splints and other appliances.

(8) Those who have undergone major surgery.

(9) Those who are unconscious or have local loss of sensation.

(10) People with arthritis who cannot move without great pain.

Areas requiring special care. Special attention should be paid to the following areas:

(1) The main pressure areas include the back of the head, elbows, buttocks, sacrum, hips, knees, ankles and heels. These are parts of the body subject to pressure because of underlying bony prominences.

(2) Any area where two skin surfaces touch: under the breasts and between the buttocks.

Effects of unrelieved pressure. The development of inflammation, noticed as redness in fair skinned races and a darker colour in dark races. If untreated this may lead to:

(1) Blistering.

(2) Breaking of the skin.

(3) Suppuration due to infection.

(4) Gangrene, that is death of the tissue.

(5) Sloughing, i.e. separation of a piece of dead tissue which can leave a cavity extending to the bone in some cases.

The earliest sign must be reported to the sister or her deputy and routine care given more frequently.

Routine care of pressure areas. Pressure areas must be relieved by every possible means for example:

(1) By changing the patient's position at least every two hours during the day and at least every four hours during the night, or more often if required by the patient's condition.

(2) By thorough bed-making to ensure smooth bottom sheets and drawsheets and by avoiding tight bedding over the body.

(3) By using appliances to minimize pressure, e.g. sorbo-rings, water pillows, special mattresses (Ripple beds), sheepskins, foam blocks, bed cradles etc.

(4) Using special care in application of splints and bandages.

(5) Ensuring that patients are not left too long on commodes and bedpans.

In addition skin must be kept scrupulously clean and dry at all times and therefore patients must be thoroughly dried after washing.

Incontinent patients must be thoroughly washed and dried and their wet clothing and bed linen changed immediately. Silicone cream may be ordered for some patients to give added protection and should be gently smoothed into the skin after careful drying.

Perspiring patients must be kept as dry as possible and their clothing changed when necessary.

Trauma to the skin must be avoided by careful lifting to avoid friction, by avoiding the wearing of rings and watches and by removing bedpans carefully.

Reddened skin must be reported immediately to the sister or her deputy.

Finally the maintenance of a well-balanced diet must be ensured, with adequate protein.

Treatment of pressure sores. As soon as the skin has become broken the ward sister will decide what treatment the patient is to have. This may include the following:

(1) The patient must be nursed if possible in a position which removes all pressure from the affected part.

(2) The sore may be covered with sterile dressings to prevent infection.

(3) A local application may be used such as bathing with an anti-septic such as Milton or Eusol, or with a healing agent such as Lotio Rubra.

(4) If infection has set in treatment will depend on bacteriological studies.

(5) A bland dressing of tulle gras may be applied.

(6) Ultraviolet light or sunbathing may be ordered.

The patient may benefit from a change of treatment from time to time, as this stimulates healing. Additional vitamins, iron and protein in the diet may also help.

Disorders of the Skin

Acne. This name is given to any inflammation of the sebaceous glands of the skin, giving rise to papules or pustules, often on the face or back, in association with adolescence or endocrine change.

Dermatitis. This term covers a number of skin conditions, caused by irritation from substances such as disinfectants, paints, detergents and acids used in the course of work, so it is usually seen on the hands.

Eczema is a very irritant condition which starts as redness followed by the formation of tiny white blisters which discharge and run together to form crusts. Some tense, nervous children are prone to it.

Impetigo is very infectious among children. It is caused by bacteria which attack the skin of poorly nourished or dirty children and is usually seen round the mouth and nose. A child with this condition should be isolated from other children on a ward.

Psoriasis shows itself as dry, scaly patches with a silvery appearance. There may be only one small patch or the whole body may be covered. The cause is unknown.

Shingles is a series of painful blisters along the course of a nerve. It is caused by a virus and is most common round the chest or over one eye.

Urticaria or nettle rash appears as large white wheals that itch intensely. It occurs in people who are sensitive to certain foods or substances.

There are no specific treatments for any of the above. Each patient is treated individually.

Poultices

Poultices provide a useful method of applying continuous heat to a part.

The kaolin poultice

A kaolin poultice retains its heat for several hours, but care must be taken in its application or serious burns may result.

Procedure. The procedure is as follows:

(1) The kaolin is heated by boiling it in its tin in a saucepan of water for about twenty minutes; the lid of the tin must first be loosened.

(2) The kaolin is spread onto a board covered with linen in a layer about 0·5 cm (0·2 in) thick.

(3) It is then covered with a single layer of gauze and carried between warmed plates to the patient's bedside.

(4) The temperature of the kaolin is tested on the back of the hand, applied gently over the affected area, covered with a warm wool and bandaged in position.

(5) Before the poultice is renewed, any dry kaolin should be removed from the skin with a swab dipped in warm olive oil. This should be carried out twelve-hourly.

After the treatment has finished the part should be kept covered with a wool bandage for a day or two.

Starch poultice

The starch poultice is useful for removing crusts in skin diseases. It should be about 2 cm (0·75 in) thick and should be left on for six to twelve hours.

Procedure. The procedure is as follows:

(1) The starch is mixed to a thick cream with a little cold water.

(2) Boiling water is stirred in and stirring continued until the starch is cool, and has become thick and jellylike.

(3) When the starch is almost cold, it is spread onto the skin, covered with a layer of old linen and bandaged in position.

Other Local Applications

Liniments are oily solutions which may contain turpentine, methyl salicylate or menthol and are warmed by standing them in hot water. They are rubbed in with the hand, after the skin has been washed, until the part is fairly dry and the skin is reddened. The gentle warmth is comforting for stiff joints and 'rheumatic' pains in muscles.

Paints, such as gentian violet, are used to control infection. They are applied to the skin with a cotton wool swab and the area is left uncovered.

Ointments are often rubbed into the skin, e.g. zinc and castor oil ointment applied to the pressure areas of an incontinent patient. Others may be applied by spreading them on strips of old linen.

Lotions may be used as wet dressings, e.g. lead lotion to reduce the swelling of a sprain. The dressing is soaked in the lotion and applied without a bandage if possible, so that evaporation takes place. See that the dressing is kept wet all the time. Other lotions, such as calamine to relieve skin irritation, are best swabbed on to the skin and left open to the air.

Nursing Care of a Patient with a Skin Disorder

It must be remembered that patients suffering from most skin conditions are not infectious. A nurse's reaction to the sight, smell or contact with these diseases could embarrass the patient, causing psychological distress which could hinder the healing process. There is no reason why these patients should not be nursed in general wards, using the general equipment. Other patients in the ward should be taught to be tolerant and understanding. It may be necessary to keep a bathroom free for the use of these patients, as many treatments involve special baths.

Patients with skin conditions may have the following:

(1) Disfigurement due to pimples, boils, scars, scaly areas.
(2) Exudates which can be very offensive.

These problems sometimes make a patient feel that he has the condition because of some misdemeanour in his past life. He feels guilty and consequently undergoes a change in personality. It is therefore the aim of the nurse to dispel all these fears, to reassure him and help him to accept and learn to live with the disfigurement. This can be achieved by not hesitating to look at or touch the part affected, by always discussing the condition in front of the patient and if an explanation is given to relatives this should be done in the presence of the patient.

Investigations. A full case history must be taken covering previous illnesses, diet, drugs, application of cosmetics, contact with detergents, etc. which may have some bearing on the problem. A full medical examination is carried out, including all parts of the body, particularly the genital area. This could be embarrassing for the patient but this can be avoided by the kind and thoughtful attitude of the nurse.

Treatment will include the relief of itching by the application of ointments and antipruritics.

Nursing measures to relieve itching must exclude excessive warmth, rough prickly clothing and emotional stress. Also idleness can contribute to increase of itching and diversional therapy may be beneficial.

Drugs may include steroids, which give relief but do not cure, antihistamines if the condition is due to an allergy and sedatives or tranquillizers to relax the patient and ensure sleep.

Ultraviolet light may help to dry the skin in some cases. Sometimes ointments are applied and covered with polythene so that they stay moist and active for a longer time.

It is important that a nurse should allow enough time to carry out the treatment correctly. If soap and water is allowed care must be taken to ensure that all the soap is rinsed off and the water changed frequently.

First Aid Treatment of Burns and Scalds

Burns are caused by dry heat, such as that from a fire, electric current or from friction.

Scalds are caused by moist heat such as boiling liquids, steam (e.g. from the spout of a kettle). It is very often forgotten that very hot water can cause a scald, even if it is not boiling.

Prevention of burns and scalds. Burns and scalds still frequently occur in spite of the many educational programmes on their prevention broadcast by radio and television and advice given to both young and old by health workers. The people who are most affected are in fact the young and elderly. It is most important that fires are not left unguarded, that electric points should be checked for faulty wiring and that boiling kettles and pans are not left unattended.

Treatment. Immediate action must be taken if a burn or scald occurs. In scalds, saturated clothing should be removed as it holds the heat, whilst in burns, flames must be smothered. The affected areas will quickly become red and inflamed, swollen and blistered if neglected. They should be cooled with cold water to relieve the pain which in turn reduces physical shock which is related to the extent of the injury and the amount of pain experienced. Shock develops as a result of fluid from the blood escaping into the tissues and thereby reducing blood volume.

It is important that the nurse should keep calm and talk to the patient. This will reassure him that he is in capable hands and that you are doing everything that you can for him.

If the burn or scald is severe the degree of shock may suddenly deepen. The best action to take is to summon an ambulance to get the patient to hospital as soon as possible and wrap him in a clean cloth or sheet. If the burn or scald is local, the part should be covered with a clean dry dressing as soon as the pain is reduced. Nothing such as ointment, should be applied to the part nor should blisters be pricked. If the nurse is at all worried the patient should be sent to his own doctor.

Most burns and scalds should receive expert medical attention as they can lead to infection and further damage.

29

The Nervous System

The nervous system controls all the other systems of the body. It is the system which so markedly distinguishes man from the rest of the animal kingdom because, compared with the size of his body, man's brain, particularly the cerebrum which deals with reasoning and memory, is very large. The brain of a medium sized dog weighs 70 g (3 oz), of a horse 270 g (9 oz) while that of a man weighs 1400 g (3 lb).

While you are reading these words your nervous system is hard at work, your eyes read and send signals to your cerebrum, your hands hold the book, you are breathing and your heart is beating. You may start to feel hungry or thirsty. Perhaps the chair you are sitting on is not comfortable and you change position because you get pins and needles in your leg. You can decide to put the book down and shut your eyes but your heart will go on beating even if you fall asleep, and if you do go to sleep a noise like a telephone ringing will awaken you. So you can see that it is possible to distinguish between two types of activities; those that you control and those that you do not, i.e. voluntary and involuntary activities.

Voluntary activities are brought about through both the central nervous system (CNS) and the peripheral nerves. It is by this means that we move the head, trunk and limbs and by which we feel sensations and see, hear and speak.

Involuntary activities are effected through the autonomic nervous system (ANS). It controls for example the movements of the involuntary muscles, in the abdominal organs and bladder, the functioning of the endocrine glands and the activities of the salivary and sweat glands.

The Central Nervous System

The central nervous system consists of the brain and the spinal cord. Both are protected against trauma; the brain lies in the skull (which except in childhood is very hard) and the spinal cord runs down the middle of the spine in the caudate canal formed by spaces in the vertebrae. In addition the brain and spinal cord are covered by three membranes called the meninges. They are the dura mater, the arachnoid mater and the pia mater. The dura mater is the outermost layer; between the arachnoid and pia mater is the subarachnoid space which is filled with a clear watery liquid called cerebrospinal fluid (CSF). This fluid cushions the brain and cord from the body cavities in which they lie.

The brain

The brain has three parts which are called the fore-brain, the hind-brain and the brain stem. Each of these consists of two areas, grey matter and white matter, all of which are encased in the hard bones

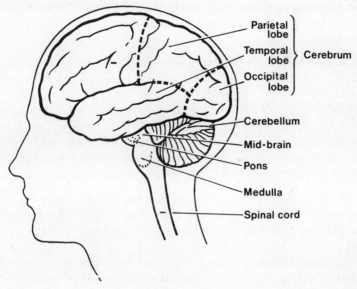

Fig. 29. The brain.

of the skull. A baby has quite a large area on top of his head where bone has not yet formed and his head must be protected from even the gentlest bumps. The grey matter which contains nerve cells and is known as the cortex makes up the outer part of the brain. White matter, the inner part, contains the nerve fibres which connect the grey matter to the body and spinal cord.

The fore-brain. Also known as the cerebrum, the fore-brain fills the vault of the skull from the level of the eyebrows to the occiput at the back. It is divided in half by a deep groove running from front to back, it is thrown into folds known as convolutions at its surface; these serve to increase the surface area and allow room for more cells. Fissures divide the cerebrum into lobes which are named according to the part of the cranium in which they lie; parietal, temporal, and occipital or frontal. The two halves or hemispheres contain spaces (ventricles) filled with CSF which acts as a water cushion for the brain and spinal cord. CSF in good health is a colourless fluid and is almost entirely, 99 per cent, water.

The cerebrum contains the centres of high intelligence such as memory and reasoning. It also contains the motor centres controlling all voluntary muscles. It receives the special sense stimuli of sight, hearing, taste, smell and touch and contains the sensory centres which give sensation to the skin and to a lesser degree to the bones, joints and muscles.

The hind-brain or cerebellum lies below the back of the cerebrum and like the cerebrum is divided into two hemispheres with finely convoluted surfaces. It helps to control balance and muscle co-ordination and tone. If it is damaged by a blow or by disease the patient is unable to stand or walk steadily but staggers. Arm and hand movements become awkward and the patient who may well be fully intelligent and aware of his condition can nevertheless not control his unsteadiness; this may be intensely distressing to him.

The brain stem. The brain stem is made up of, at the top, the mid-brain, below it the pons and below that the medulla oblongata. The brain stem lies between and links the cerebrum and the spinal cord.

The pons is a bridge between the two hemispheres of the cerebellum which it joins to the medulla oblongata. It consists almost entirely of white matter.

The medulla is a small bulb-like structure which links the brain to the spinal cord with which it is continuous. It also contains in its grey matter the vital centres controlling the heart and circulation, breathing, the movements of the stomach and intestines and the secretion of digestive juices. In the medulla oblongata most of the motor fibres cross over from one side to the other with the result that the left side of the brain controls the right side of the body and the right side of the brain the left side of the body. The medulla also contains the reflex centres which control the reflex actions of swallowing, vomiting, coughing and sneezing. These are all actions which occur without our deliberate thought.

The spinal cord

About as thick as one's little finger the spinal cord comes from the medulla oblongata and runs down the spinal canal for 38–45 cm (18 in approx.) to the base of the first lumbar vertebra; it ends in a bunch of nerves called the cauda equina.

Like the medulla the cord consists of white matter on its surface and grey matter in the centre. (You will remember that in the cerebrum the grey matter is outside to give plenty of area for nerve cells, with the fibres or white matter inside. In the spinal cord the fibres must be on the outside so that they can connect up to the muscles and sensory nerve endings via the peripheral nerves.)

The Peripheral Nerves

The peripheral nerves arise from the brain and the spinal cord. There are forty-three pairs altogether. Twelve pairs of cranial nerves arise from the brain and thirty-one pairs of spinal nerves arise from the spinal cord. Messages from the brain pass down the spinal cord, via the peripheral nerves *to* the tissues. Messages *from* the tissues are returned in a similar way via the peripheral nerves to the spinal cord and brain.

The Autonomic Nervous System

This supplies nerves to the internal organs and blood vessels. It is mostly concerned with sending instructions *from* the brain and is better supplied with efferent (outgoing) fibres than with afferent (inward) ones. This explains why internal organs are not very sensitive to pain and why a disease may progress a long way before we become aware of it.

The autonomic nervous system consists of (1) the sympathetic nerves (2) the parasympathetic nerves. Both sets of nerves work to counter each other's actions.

The sympathetic nerves prepare the individual for response to an emergency situation, that is to say for fight or flight. Sudden fear makes the heart beat faster to send more oxygen-rich blood out to the muscles to prepare them for action. However a stomach full of food is no help in an emergency so the flow of digestive juices stops and you may feel sick and even vomit.

The parasympathetic nerves react to pleasant emotions so that a happy and relaxed person's digestion works well and his heart beat and breathing are steady. This is why it is very important for your patients to be carefully and kindly nursed.

The autonomic nervous system being responsible for involuntary activity reacts to insults to the body. Therefore a surgeon operates as gently and quickly as he can; even so after an abdominal operation a patient may for several days suffer from constipation because peristalsis has stopped.

Nerve Tissue

Nerve tissue consists of nerve cells and nerve fibres. Each cell has one long fibre, the axon and several short fibres called dendrites. The cell and its fibres form a neurone which is the basic unit of the nervous system.

Neurones carry impulses:

(1) Out from the brain: efferent neurones.
(2) Towards the brain: afferent neurones.
(3) In the brain and spinal cord thus linking efferent and afferent neurones: connector or association neurones.

The Reflex Arc

Reflex actions take place without reference to the brain at all through what is called a reflex arc. Sudden heat or a pinprick produces a very quick automatic response. You do not have to think about taking your hand from under a stream of scalding water; it snatches away almost before you feel the heat. In fact your muscles get the signal before your brain does. The route for the signal is from the nerve ending in the skin to the CNS (usually the spine) then to both the appropriate motor neurone and the brain. The motor neurone activates the muscle while the signal is still going by the other nerves to the brain. This saves time and is a form of safety device. It may well be that after all, the water is not too hot to touch and from your cerebrum your conscious or deliberate decision may be to put your hand under the tap again. This time because you have had time to decide you will be able to hold your hand there and the reflex action will not occur.

Disorders of the Nervous System

When any part of the nervous system is damaged by injury or disease the result can be seen in the person's behaviour or in the effect on some part of the body. A broken back and therefore severed spinal cord will cause paralysis. Damage to the brain may result in loss of speech or in imbecility. Prenatal damage or imperfect development of the fetus can result in permanent mental or physical handicap.

Cerebrovascular accident (CVA)

More ordinarily known as a stroke, CVA results in sudden loss of consciousness or in paralysis of one side or part of one side of the body. Rare in young people but one of the most common conditions encountered among older patients, CVA is the result of a blood vessel in the brain bursting or becoming blocked by an embolus. On recovering consciousness the patient may be unable to speak or move some of his limbs, an experience particularly terrifying because of its totally unexpected occurrence.

The nurse must behave kindly to her patient, speaking to him though he may be unable to reply. Speech therapy may be needed and the occupational therapist plays a very important part in the patient's recovery. Medical treatment for this condition is virtually unknown and it is the patient's own determination and the quality of nursing which may decide on the degree of recovery.

Epilepsy

Many cases of epilepsy may be detected but seldom cured though the symptoms may be suppressed with drugs. The epileptic fit, *grand mal*, is broadly in three stages. At first the eyes stare, the teeth are clenched and the subject becomes stiff. Then follow violent convulsions during which the patient may injure himself and lastly the patient falls into a deep sleep. On waking the epileptic may be very confused and quite often in a towering rage, resenting any help or kindness offered.

Petit mal is a mild form of epilepsy seen sometimes in children who in class develop a blank stare for a few seconds and total unawareness of their surroundings; rarely will they fall to the ground.

An epileptic person when in a fit must have his false teeth removed if possible though he may inadvertently bite the helping hand. He need not be physically restrained though dangerous obstacles should be kept out of his reach.

Meningitis

This illness, inflammation of the meninges, is caused by bacterial or viral infection. It is more common in children than in adults and its onset is sudden, with vomiting, dislike of light (photophobia), headache and marked stiffness of the neck. As the disease progresses the head is retracted and the back arched. Lumbar puncture will enable the causative organism to be identified and the appropriate drug prescribed.

Brain tumours

Tumours in the brain can be benign, that is to say encapsulated and not likely to recur if removed, or malignant which means free to spread. Quite apart from damage to the part of the brain in which they occur tumours cause marked distress by raising the pressure within the skull. Symptoms include agonizing headache, vomiting, blindness and unconsciousness.

Treatment of a brain tumour is either by surgery or by radiotherapy or both.

Infantile paralysis (poliomyelitis)

Acute anterior poliomyelitis is inflammation of the anterior horn cells of the spinal cord. It is more common in children and young adults than in older people but is one of the diseases now rarely encountered because of immunization by the vaccine devised by Dr Salk. The virus which gives rise to the infection enters the body by way of the intestines. The degree of plegia or paresis varies but if the respiratory muscles are affected the patient must be nursed with a respirator.

Parkinson's disease (paralysis agitans)

This is the most common neurological disease in the elderly. It usually starts between the ages of fifty and sixty and shows as tremor, stiffness of the body and slowness of movement. In addition the face may become masklike, though when the sufferer smiles the smile may remain for many seconds. Walking becomes ungainly, and having started to move the patient may find it impossible to stop. Remember that the patient may look stupid and be unable to speak intelligently. Mentally he is perfectly normal athough his condition is very likely to cause acute depression.

Multiple sclerosis

This is a disease of temperate rather than tropical climates though the reason for this distribution is not known. It is more common in women than in men and may start as early as the twentieth year. It is what is called a demyelinating disease; the myelin sheath of nerve fibres is destroyed rather as though the insulation were being stripped off an electrical flex. It is progressive and incurable, though the rate of its progress varies and there may be long periods of remission giving false hope of cure.

Symptoms include blurring of vision and painful eye movement, loss of control of hand and tingling, stiffness or heaviness in a limb. Walking becomes slower and more awkward, speech is slurred. There is a steady slow decline into permanent bedcare.

Cerebral palsy

This is a condition which is incurable but not progressive. Present at birth it is caused by damage to brain cells which control the muscles. The child cannot make co-ordinate movements because he has no control over his limbs which are stiff and ungainly. The term 'spastic' is used to describe these children, who may be highly intelligent. Speech therapy and physiotherapy may produce great improvement.

Paralysis and paresis

Plegia is the technical term used for paralysis and means loss of power. With a prefix it indicates the area affected as follows:

(1) Monoplegia: Paralysis of one limb (arm or leg).
(2) Paraplegia: Paralysis of both legs.
(3) Hemiplegia: Paralysis of one side of the body.
(4) Quadriplegia: Paralysis of all four limbs.
(5) Ophthalmoplegia: Paralysis of eye movement.

Paresis means weakness and is also used with a prefix, i.e., para-paresis. Plegia and paresis are caused by damage in the skull (CVA, tumour or birth injury) or by injury or disease in the spinal cord.

The Neurological Patient

It is in the care of the patient with a neurological condition that nursing reaches its peak of responsibility and achievement. The unconscious patient can very easily be injured by incorrect (not necessarily careless) handling; the conscious but immobilized patient needs reassurance and encouragement.

The patient may be unconscious or in other ways unable to give any history of his illness and anyone who has accompanied him to hospital must be asked for help. Relatives will be distressed and you must be ready to listen to what they want to say and to tell the doctor anything which will help in his diagnosis. Headaches, vomiting, visual disturbance or spells of dizziness are particularly important. In epilepsy an examination will reveal nothing though the history will provide the diagnosis.

In addition to the usual recording of temperatures, pulse and respiration the following must be observed and accurately recorded by the nurse as soon as possible:

(1) Head: Patient conscious or unconscious?
             Headache: Frequency and severity,

(2) Eyes: Can the patient see?
             Do his eyelids droop?
             Are the pupils dilated or contracted and of equal size?
             Does he try to avoid the light?
             Are his eyes his own? Look for artificial eye or cosmetic contact lens.

(3) Ears: Can he hear you?
             Discharge: Note amount and colour.

(4) Speech: Clear or slurred?
             Stammer.
             Use of wrong words.

(5) Gait: If he is walking, is he steady? Is there any tremor?

These are all points to be noted by the nurse. The detailed neurological examination is carried out by the physician and for this he will need a tray or trolley with a number of articles each chosen for a specific test.

The examination trolley: The following articles are required:

To test the eyes: ophthalmoscope, red-headed and white-headed pins, torch and reading charts.

To test the ears: auroscope, noise box and tuning forks.

To test the nose: bottles of: oil of cloves, oil of peppermint, ginger, coffee and aniseed.

To test the tongue: bottle of: saline, quinine, citric acid and syrup.

To test sensation: hot water, cold water, cotton wool, wooden blocks, orange sticks, pins, patella hammer, tape measure, 2 pt discriminator, spirit lamp and laryngeal mirrors.

In addition a doctor may like to have a number of everyday objects such as a pen, buttons and paperclip to test the patient's powers of recognition and description and in case the doctor wants to see the patient standing out of bed, a dressing-gown, slippers and examination pants must be at hand.

The nurse's two duties are to help the doctor and to encourage and support the patient.

Lumbar puncture

A lumbar puncture is a means of gaining access to the CSF for diagnostic or therapeutic purposes. (Two other methods rarely used are by cisternal puncture and by direct entry into the ventricles via a burr hole in the skull.)

For diagnostic purposes:

(1) The doctor can measure the pressure of CSF, note its colour and send a specimen to be examined in the pathology department.

(2) An X-ray opaque substance or air may be inserted to reveal a spinal lesion.

For therapeutic purposes:

(1) To administer a curative drug, e.g. penicillin.

(2) To induce anaesthesia when a general anaesthesia is contra-indicated.

Procedure. The procedure is as follows: An aseptic technique is essential to reduce the risk of introducing infection and ideally the patient is wheeled in his bed to a treatment room where privacy, better lighting and a cleaner working area exist. The patient's co-operation is needed and he must be kept as comfortable and still as possible. The doctor may prescribe a sedative.

The patient is placed on his left side with his back at the edge of the bed and with his hips and knees flexed at ninety degrees; he must not be left unattended or he might fall backwards off the bed. Plastic and drawsheets are placed under the patient's back to protect his own sheets. Doctor and nurse each wear a mask and the doctor puts on his gloves and swabs the patient's lumbar area. The patient is warned that he is to have a local anaesthetic and the nurse opens the local anaesthetic packet for the doctor to remove the syringe. Both check that the anaesthetic is the correct one and the doctor injects a small amount into several places over the intended site, that is to say over the area between lumbar vertebrae 3 and 4 or 4 and 5. Some time must be allowed for the anaesthetic to take effect and during this time the patient is reassured. He, you must remember, can see nothing of what is going on.

When the doctor is ready he inserts the lumbar puncture needle and CSF drips out. The two-way tap and manometer are attached to the needle. All this time the nurse looks after the patient and encourages him to lie still. By holding his hand and watching his face she can at once detect any pain or anxiety. Once pressures have been recorded the doctor turns the two-way tap so that CSF drains into the specimen pots held in position; three specimens are taken and labelled 1, 2, and 3. The manometer is disconnected, the needle is pulled quickly out and the puncture sealed with colloidion or an Elastoplast dressing.

Care of the patient after lumbar puncture. The patient is made comfortable and advised to lie flat for twenty-four hours. This helps to prevent headache which often follows lumbar puncture as a result of the change of pressure of CSF. A salty diet and increased fluid intake hasten the replacement of CSF and a mild analgesic may be prescribed. The patient's condition must be watched and changes reported at once.

Nursing care of the unconscious patient

When a patient is unconscious he loses his protective senses and is no longer aware of his surroundings. His condition calls for the highest skills and at all times the nurse must remember that the patient is a human being and should be treated with respect. She takes care not to expose the patient while she is attending to him and she must anticipate his needs.

Arrival in the ward. A very experienced nurse will always be present when an unconscious patient is admitted to the ward and her first responsibility is to ensure that the patient's airway remains clear. This she does by placing the patient either in the semiprone or in the lateral position. Both of these positions reduce the risk of the patient's tongue falling back into the pharynx, and they enable secretions to drain from the mouth. Dentures, which might become dislodged, are removed and the patency of the airway is ensured in addition by cleaning the nostrils if necessary.

The patient's position is changed at regular intervals of two hours to prevent lung collapse and the development of pressure sores. Two nurses are required for this and the interval of two hours must be strictly adhered to; the unconscious patient can always be left for just a few more minutes so that two hours becomes two and a quarter and then two and a half and so on. A pillow placed behind the patient will stop him rolling onto his back and another between his legs will prevent them rubbing each other.

The patient's toilet

The skin. A daily blanket bath is given in addition to any other washing required. The patient's skin is examined for sore places or cracks and to determine that it remains generally healthy and supple.

The mouth. An unconscious person cannot take anything by mouth. Therefore his salivary glands are not stimulated and his mouth and tongue become dry and in time sore and cracked. Pathogenic micro-organisms may easily cause infection which can spread to all parts of the respiratory and alimentary tracts; by way of the Eustachian tubes the infection can reach the middle ear and via the bony sinuses, the brain. Liquid paraffin applied to the lips and tongue prevents cracking, and the mouth is cleaned with a mouthwash solution on a gauze swab firmly secured to mouth forceps.

The eyes. Sometimes an unconscious patient's eyes remain open and have to be held closed with Sellotape. The blinking reflex which spreads moisture over the surface of the eye will be absent and dust and the patient's own hair entering his eyes cause irritation and inflammation. His eyes must be kept clear of the pillow and the doctor may order drops of liquid paraffin to be administered at least twice a day to keep the eyes moist. Other eye care is performed three-hourly.

The ears. Discharge from the ears must be reported at once because it may be CSF from the subarachnoid space. Mopping up the discharge must be an aseptic technique because infection can enter directly to the meninges, spinal cord and brain at the point where CSF is leaking.

The bladder. The patient can be incontinent of urine for either of two reasons; he may be unable to retain it in the bladder in the normal way or he may have retention which distends the bladder to such an extent that urine dribbles out. The doctor may suggest catheterization which is an aseptic procedure and at the same time prescribe antibiotic cover or an urinary antiseptic to prevent infection.

The bowels. Constipation is common though daily evacuation is not necessary and an aperient may be prescribed after two or three days. If the aperient is not effective two glycerine suppositories may be given. Faecal incontinence with overflow can resemble diarrhoea.

Feeding. The unconscious patient cannot eat and must be fed by means of an oesophageal tube which is normally passed through the nose, down the oesophagus to the stomach. It is quite easy to insert the tube into the lungs instead of the stomach and there are two simple ways of ensuring that it does arrive in the right place.

In one method a little of the stomach content is withdrawn and tested for acidity by placing a drop of it on blue litmus paper which should turn red; if the litmus does not turn red it is very unlikely that the tube is in the stomach.

For the second method two nurses are needed. One attaches a syringe containing 5 ml of air to the end of the naso-oesophageal tube and injects air down it while the other listens to the stomach with a stethoscope.

The tube's position must be checked before every feed by a third method. The funnel and tube through which the feed is to be given can be connected to the naso-oesophageal tube and the funnel held upside down under water. A stream of bubbles indicates that the end of the tube is in the airway but if there are none or only one or two bubbles the end of the tube must be in the stomach.

Physiotherapy. The physiotherapist gives passive movements to the patient's limbs to prevent them from becoming stiff and it is quite usual for a nurse to do this between visits by the physiotherapist.

30

The Special Senses

To keep us informed about our surroundings we are provided with a number of detectors called the special senses. These pass information to the brain so that we can take action to avoid danger, recognize friends and move about with confidence. Our senses therefore detect those things which naturally affect us and these include light, sound, smell, taste and people, animals and objects with which we come into contact. If this sounds childishly obvious consider for a moment what we cannot detect, radioactivity, carbon monoxide gas, ultraviolet light and very low and very high frequency sounds. These can cause us real damage and, if we suffer their effects for too long, death.

Our senses have developed so as to be most useful to us as human beings. Other creatures in other surroundings develop their senses in different ways. The dog has a refined sense of smell, the hawk finer eyesight than we have and the bat a wonderfully acute sense of hearing.

We all use our senses automatically and a nurse is trained to use them deliberately to help her to nurse her patients. She sees the colour, hears the wheezing breath and feels the hot skin of the feverish patient.

The Eye

Structure
The eyes are the organs which transmit light signals to the brain. They are suspended by ligaments in holes in the skull called orbits and can be turned in various directions by muscles attached to the outside of the eyeball. The eyeball has three distinct layers:

(1) Sclera – the white of the eye, transparent at the front to allow light to enter, where it is called the cornea. This completely covers the inner layers.

(2) Choroid, ciliary body and iris. These comprise the vascular and pigmented middle layer which is non-reflecting so that light which enters the eye is totally absorbed. At the front of the eye is the iris,

coloured brown, green, blue or grey, which is the aperture which by expansion or contraction controls the amount of light reaching the lens to be focussed on the retina.

(3) Retina. The layer of nerve endings which detect the light and transmit impulses to the optic centre in the brain.

To reach the retina light passes through the conjunctiva, the cornea, the aqueous humour, the lens, and lastly the vitreous humour which fills the inner part of the eye.

Note. The pupil is not a structure but a hole in the choroid; it appears black because no light is reflected out of it from the retina.

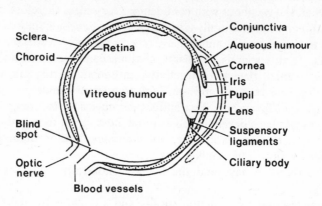

Fig. 30. The eye.

Protection

The eyes are protected from injury by being located in the strong bone orbits; the tops of the orbits, the brows, also shade them from the light. The eyelids are lined with mucous membrane which turns back (reflects) over the eye; this is the conjunctiva which forms sacs above and below the eye.

The lacrimal glands situated on the upper and outer margins of the eyes, provide tear fluid to wash over the eye. This drains into the nasolacrimal duct and into the nose. Tear fluid keeps the eye clean, acts also as a lubricant and contains an antibacterial compound called lysozyme. When we are very sad or happy the lacrimal glands produce so much fluid that the eye overflows and tears run down our cheeks.

The eyelashes prevent the entry of dust and also when we screw up our eyes help shade them against bright light.

Focusing

The eye gives the brain a clear sharp picture of our surroundings and we can see things close to us as clearly as we see things far away. There are limits to this ability and you can prove this to yourself by bringing this book closer and closer to your eyes until you can no longer see the firm outlines of the letters. The blurring of the letters arises from the inability of the lens to cope with the extreme situation. You will also see two pages instead of one because each eye sends its own picture at this distance whereas at usual distances the eyes combine to send the same message to the brain.

Focusing is possible because the lens can be made to change shape; the closer the page the rounder the lens becomes. It is not really sensible to compare the eye to a camera because a camera lens does not change shape but moves nearer to or further from the film.

The lens is held in position by suspensory ligaments which are themselves also attached to the ciliary muscle. It is the contraction inwards of this muscle, a squeezing effect, which causes the lens to fatten to focus on nearby objects. This explains why the eyes become tired by close work such as reading or needlework. As is the case with any muscle the ciliary muscle becomes fatigued and must be given time to recover.

Ophthalmic Nursing

Preoperative care

Blind people are almost always cheerful and self-reliant because they have learnt to compensate for their loss of sight by placing more reliance on their other senses. The patient who is shortly to undergo eye surgery will not have made these compensations and will be anxious not only about having the operation but about its outcome. It is therefore highly desirable that he is admitted to hospital a day or two before the operation so that he becomes accustomed to the ward environment and gets to know the staff upon whom he will have to rely. During this period he can be taught the breathing and leg exercises he will have to do after his operation and to use a feeding cup.

Postoperative care

The eye cannot be immobilized like a leg or arm in plaster and the patient has therefore to provide immobilization himself. He is nursed sitting up with his head well supported by pillows and is given food which needs little chewing; he is not allowed to become constipated and any sign of coughing is dealt with promptly.

It is quite usual for the patient to be allowed no visitors for two or three days and when they are allowed kissing may be forbidden in case the eye is knocked. The nurse herself has to take great care never to startle the patient but speak so that he knows where she is. She naturally tells him what she is about to do when tidying his bed-clothes and when washing him.

Ophthalmic nursing procedures

Instillation of drops. Eyedrops and ointments used in the ophthalmic ward may be classified as follows:

(1) Antibiotics.
(2) Miotics, i.e. pupil contractors.
(3) Mydriatics, i.e. pupil dilators.
(4) Steroids, i.e. anti-inflammatory drugs.
(5) Local anaesthetics.
(6) Those for diagnosis.
(7) Artificial tears.

These are liquids which are instilled into the eye. As with all drug administering, two nurses check the drug, dosage and time with the prescription sheet.

Procedure. The procedure is as follows:

(1) The patient who may be lying down or sitting is asked to tilt his head back and to look up.
(2) The lower lid is gently pulled down to evert it.
(3) From about 2 cm (1 in) above the eye the drop is instilled into the lower fornix.

Note: Do not touch the eyelashes with the dropper as this will contaminate it.

When anaesthetizing the cornea the drop is allowed to fall onto or just above the cornea so that the fluid flows over its surface.

Irrigation. This is done, frequently as an emergency, to neutralize an acid or caustic alkaline in the eye and also to remove a foreign body; it is also used to cleanse the eye of a patient with purulent conjunctivitis. When a caustic fluid has entered the eye, speed and copious use of water (tap water is perfectly suitable) take precedence over the niceties of ideal sterile procedures. Any clean vessel such as a teacup will serve for immediate action.

In a less hectic situation use an undine filled with warmed normal saline and test its temperature by pouring a little onto the patient's cheek. The rate of flow is controlled by placing a finger over the hole in the side of the undine.

Taking a conjunctival specimen : Requirements. These are as follows:

Culture plate.
Spirit lamp and box of matches.
Platinum loop.
Gauze swabs.

Procedure. The procedure is as follows:

(1) Explain the procedure to the patient who is placed in a comfortable position.

(2) Put on a face mask and wash the hands.

(3) Heat the platinum wire in the spirit lamp's flame (it will cool completely in ten seconds).

(4) Expose the lower fornix and ask the patient to look up.

(5) Stroke the platinum loop along the lower fornix and immediately over the surface of the culture plate.

(6) Replace the lid of the culture plate.

(7) Heat platinum loop to sterilize it.

(8) Send culture plate and request form to the pathology laboratory.

Note: Take particular care that the loop touches only the lower fornix and not the eyelashes.

An alternative method is to use a sterile swab in a sterile test tube instead of a platinum loop.

Cutting eyelashes. The patient is placed in a comfortable position so that he can keep his head still. The nurse applies petroleum jelly to the upper blade of the scissors, the patient closes his eyes and the nurse with her hand resting comfortably cuts along the top lashes with a single cut. The cut lashes stick to the petroleum jelly which is wiped off the blade before the next cut. When the lower eyelashes are being cut the lower lid is gently pulled down while the patient looks upwards.

The eyes are then cleaned with normal saline.

Hot steam bathing. This simple procedure is used to ease the irritation caused by conjunctivitis, blepharitis (inflammation of the eyelids) or by a stye. A wooden spoon is covered with lint held in place by a piece of cotton bandage. The patient dips the spoon into a bowl of boiling hot water and holds it under his eye so that the steam rises and warms it. The wad of material must not touch the eye. The patient continues until in a few minutes the water cools.

Disorders of the eye

Cataract is a condition in which the lens becomes cloudy and ultimately opaque. Treatment is always surgical. In children the lens is incised so that the lens fluid enters and mixes with the aqueous humour and will be absorbed. For elderly patients the treatment is complete removal of the lens, which therefore results in blindness in that eye. Blindness would in any event be caused by the cataract. Preoperative treatment will include the instillation of mydriatic drops approximately every fifteen minutes; the exact timing will be decided by the surgeon.

Glaucoma. Increased pressure of the aqueous humour inside the eye which is usually very painful will lead to permanent loss of vision if untreated. The glaucoma patient is usually admitted as an emergency and treatment to reduce tension is started at once. This includes intravenous or intramuscular administration of a diuretic, intensive treatment with miotics and suitable analgesia. The patient will often be generally ill and vomiting but it is the eye pain that indicates glaucoma and not an abdominal disorder.

Squint. The patient, usually a child, is admitted from the waiting list. His eyelashes are trimmed after he has been anaesthetized. He can be sent home possibly only two days after the operation.

Ophthalmia neonatorum is an infection of the eyes of the newborn baby. It is treated with antibiotics and the baby's eyes are cleaned to remove the pus which is formed.

Styes are due to infection of an eye lash follicle. Steam bathing or removal of the lash usually effect a cure.

Systemic ophthalmic signs. The eyes may show evidence of a general infection elsewhere in the body and the nurse too must always report any unhealthy appearance, redness for instance, of the eyes.

The Ear

The ear serves two very vital functions. It enables us to detect sound and it gives us our sense of balance; it is divided into three separate areas:

(1) The external ear. These are the visible parts, called the auricle and the external auditory meatus which is the funnel-shaped tube leading inwards. At the end of this tube is the eardrum or tympanic membrane.

(2) The middle ear. This is a cavity in the bone immediately inside the eardrum. It is connected to the upper part of the nose by the Eustachian tube which admits air to the cavity and ensures that the air pressure on either side of the eardrum is equal.

(3) The internal ear. Also known as the labyrinth, it is made up of cavities and tubes called the semicircular canals. In one part, the cochlea, is the organ of Corti which provides the connections to the auditory nerves.

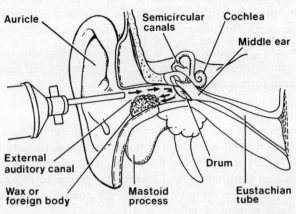

Fig. 31. The ear, showing position of syringe for removal of a foreign body.

Sound and hearing

Sound is vibration which can be felt or detected by the ear. Usually it is carried by the air but it is also conducted by water and by most solids such as waterpipes or railway lines. In outer space where there is no air to carry the sound no noises can be heard. Human beings can detect air vibrations between approximately fifteen per second, very low notes and 20 000 per second, very high notes. As we grow older the range we hear decreases, particularly in the high notes.

Balance

This is provided by the semicircular canals, the saccule and the utricle in the internal ear which both contain endolymph; changes in the attitude of the head and movement cause changes in the pressure of the endolymph on the nerve fibres.

Injury to the inner ear will affect balance and very rarely congenital malformation may result not only in total deafness but in a complete lack of the sense of balance so that the sufferer can only walk about in daylight where vertical lines provided by buildings enable him to remain upright.

Disorders of the ear

Otitis media. Inflammation of the middle ear arises from an infection spreading up the Eustachian tube. The patient may be feverish and feel pain and become slightly deaf. Treatment of the nasal infection may be sufficient though the physician may immediately prescribe antibiotic therapy.

Mastoiditis. Nowadays this is rarely seen, being an extension of otitis media. Symptoms of otitis media are increased and surgery may be required to remove a mastoid abscess.

Syringing the ear

The eardrum is very sensitive and delicate; therefore ear syringing to remove a foreign body or wax must be done extremely carefully and only on the instructions of a doctor. The solution used is made up of sodium bicarbonate and glycerine together forming approximately a quarter of the total mixture. Alternatively warm olive oil may be used instead of sodium bicarbonate.

The syringe is held in both hands, one resting against the patient's head to prevent the nozzle entering the meatus too far. The tip of the nozzle should be only just within the meatus to direct the stream of solution along the top of it to drive wax out along its lower length.

The deaf patient

The deaf or partially deaf patient is isolated from all the incidental friendly sounds and can become very lonely even in a crowd. Before talking to someone with poor hearing attract his attention, otherwise the first he hears is a raised and impatient voice shouting from an angry face. Also look directly at your patient because your lip movements will help him to understand you.

The Nose

The nose contains the nerve endings which provide the sense of smell. This sense rapidly becomes insensitive which means that if for example you smell household gas when you go into a house or room and suspect a gas leak, you must not assume that the gas has dispersed if you can no longer smell it a few seconds later. You must open windows and doors to make sure that the gas is at least diluted.

Socially we have become very smell conscious and any natural body smell is considered offensive. Nevertheless the nose is a sensitive detector of bad living conditions, bad drainage and of atmospheric pollution. Both smoking and snuff-taking blunt the sense of smell but sniffing increases the flow to the top of the nasal passage which is where the nerve endings of smell are situated.

The Tongue

The tongue is the organ of taste and can detect only sweetness, saltiness, acidity and bitterness. The other flavours are detected by the nose and this explains why people with a cold (coryza) or hay fever cannot taste their food properly. The tongue helps in swallowing and chewing and with the roof of the mouth plays an important role in speech.

31

Hormones

The human body which is itself a collection of very complex chemical compounds is controlled in two ways. Firstly by the nervous system which is electrical in character and secondly by the endocrine system which is chemical.

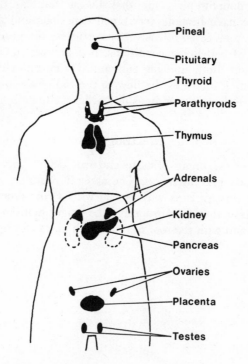

Fig. 32. The endocrine glands and other organs which secrete hormones.

Within the head, neck and body are a number of glands which take chemicals from the blood stream to make a series of special compounds called hormones. These hormones are secreted into the blood stream and carried by it all round the body. Each hormone has an effect on one or several organs or tissues and in some cases on the other glands as well.

Some organs have an endocrine function and some glands produce chemicals which are not hormones. The ovaries produce ova and the female sex hormones, the kidneys produce hormones as well as being high pressure filters, the placenta nourishes the fetus by transfer of oxygen and nutriments from the mother and also manufactures a number of hormones.

The rate at which a gland secretes hormones is not constant but varies according to the requirements of organs and tissues for those hormones. When sufficient has been produced for a particular purpose a second hormone serves as a messenger to instruct the gland to slow down production, a process known as negative feedback.

The pituitary gland

Through its hormones the pituitary gland influences the activity of the other endocrine glands and it is for this reason looked upon as the master of the endocrine orchestra. It is situated in the base of the brain in the sella turcica and has two parts, an anterior lobe and a posterior lobe. The anterior lobe produces several hormones the most important being the following:

Growth hormone (GH) affects the growth of bone and muscle and determines the size of each of us. Oversecretion in childhood causes gigantism and in adults causes acromegaly, a condition in which there is excessive growth of the bones of the lower jaw, the hands and the feet. Undersecretion in children results in dwarfism.

Thyroid stimulating hormone (TSH) stimulates the activity of the thyroid gland.

Adrenocorticotrophic hormone (ACTH) stimulates the cortex of the adrenal gland to produce hormones.

Follicle stimulating hormone (FSH). In the female this hormone affects the development of the ovarian follicles; in the male it stimulates sperm cell production in the testes.

Luteinizing hormone (LH). In the female it affects the corpus luteum and in the male stimulates the production of testosterone in the testes.

Lactogenic hormone. After the mother has given birth this hormone stimulates the secretory cells in the breast to produce milk.

The posterior lobe secretes two hormones:

Oxytocin. In labour the muscles of the uterus only are made to contract first to expel the baby and then to dislodge the placenta after the baby has been born.

Antidiuretic hormone (ADH) or vasopressin concentrates the urine by increasing the amount of fluid absorbed by the kidneys. It also raises the blood pressure.

The thyroid gland

The two lobes of the thyroid gland are situated on either side of the trachea and joined across the front of it by a narrow isthmus. The gland secretes two hormones which are involved in the general metabolism of the body, in other words the rate at which the body lives; these are thyroxine and triiodothyroxine and both contain a high proportion of iodine.

Goitre. Enlargement of the thyroid gland, may occur in districts whose water and food lack iodine. The condition is now prevented by adding iodine to the water supply or to cooking salt.

Cretinism. Undersecretion results in the child becoming a cretin, i.e. a mentally retarded dwarf with a broad face and large mouth.

Myxoedema. In adults undersecretion causes mental slowness and physical idleness, the patient's temperature is low, the skin becomes dry and the hair lank and coarse.

Thyrotoxicosis (Graves' disease) is a condition in which oversecretion produces a clear picture of irritability, loss of weight, rapid pulse and protruding eyeballs, all signs of increased metabolic rate. The skin is moist and the patient may be in a highly nervous state and very difficult to manage.

The adrenal glands

Approximately 2·5 cm (1 in) long the adrenal (or suprarenal) glands are situated over each kidney. They have a very rich blood supply and network of nerves of the sympathetic part of the automatic nervous system and are therefore closely involved in emotional disturbances. Each gland has two parts, a cortex and a medulla. The adrenal cortex secretes a group of chemicals called corticoids whose functions are explained by their names:

(1) Glucocorticoids are concerned with metabolism of proteins, carbohydrates and fats.

(2) Mineralocorticoids control the kidney tubules so as to secrete excess potassium and to retain sodium and chloride in the body.

(3) Sex corticoids affect the development and function of the gonads and also the temperament of both male and female.

The adrenal medulla secretes adrenaline and noradrenaline. Adrenaline increases the metabolic rate when an emergency arises as follows. Adrenaline:

(1) Releases as glucose, glycogen stored in the liver.

(2) Contracts the arterioles in the skin and internal organs.

(3) Dilates the bronchial tubes to increase oxygen intake.

These three effects concentrate the blood supply in the muscles, including the heart and enrich the blood with glucose and oxygen. We are prepared to flee or fight and the pallor of the skin of the face is a readily visible sign that the blood is being used elsewhere.

Noradrenaline contracts the blood vessels and thereby raises the blood pressure.

Cushing's syndrome. Oversecretion of hydrocortisone from the adrenal cortex causes obesity, diabetes, hypertension and osteoporosis. The patient's face becomes fat and round and there is excessive growth of hair on the face and body.

Addison's disease. Undersecretion from the adrenal cortex causes low blood pressure, low blood sugar and weakness of the muscles. The skin becomes bronzed and if this is evenly spread the patient may appear to have a healthy suntan.

The parathyroid glands

These are two pairs of glands situated behind each half of the thyroid. They secrete parathormone which controls calcium metabolism. Oversecretion results in calcium being extracted from the bones, causing osteitis fibrosa and being returned to the blood and urine. The increase in calcium may result in renal calculi or stones. Undersecretion causes muscular spasms, tetany.

The gonads

The ovaries produce:

Oestrogen which is concerned with the regulation of menstruation and with the secondary sex characteristics.
Progesterone which is involved in the preparation of the uterus for the reception of the fertilized ovum.

The testes secrete hormones called androgens, the principal one being testosterone. This causes the changes which occur at puberty, deepening of the voice and the growth of hair on the face and body.

The kidneys

The hormone erythropoietin is secreted by the kidney and stimulates the bone marrow to produce red blood cells.

The pancreas

The islets of Langerhans scattered thoughout the pancreas secrete insulin which metabolizes sucrose to glucose. Deficiency of insulin causes diabetes mellitus.

The thymus gland

The function of this gland is not fully understood though it appears to be involved with immunity. It decreases in size after puberty and if removed from patients with myasthenia gravis appears to have a beneficial effect.

The pineal gland

The pineal gland too has no known purpose but it provides in the adult a useful reference point in X-ray examination of the brain; it becomes calcified and therefore opaque to X-rays.

Endocrine Emergencies

The commonly met emergencies which arise from malfunction of one or more of the endocrine glands are the following:

(1) Hyperglycaemic, or diabetic coma.
(2) Hypoglycaemic coma.
(3) Thyroid crisis.

Many of the illnesses which arise from oversecretion or undersecretion of a hormone are long drawn out, perhaps over many years and treatment also is usually over a long period. However three emergency conditions call for immediate action if the patient is not to suffer permanent damage or death.

Hyperglycaemic coma is a coma caused by the body's inability to absorb glucose, therefore the brain is starved of the nourishment which is in the blood but which the body cannot use. Administration of insulin will enable the patient to metabolize sucrose to glucose and the comatose state will be alleviated.

Hypoglycaemic coma is caused by lack of available sugar in a diabetic patient who has already taken insulin. The patient is given sugar by mouth which the insulin converts to glucose. Diabetic patients are advised to carry a few lumps of sugar with them so that when they feel that a coma is imminent they can prevent it by eating some. A doctor may find it necessary to administer glucose intravenously.

Thyroid crisis may arise after a complete or partial thyroidectomy. The patient's metabolism increases and may be seen in a raised temperature, general excitability and in a faster pulse; the cause is excessive secretion of thyroxine and treatment is by drugs, cortisone or digitalis for instance.

Suggested Further Reading

There is a natural temptation when you start nursing to try to absorb a great deal of information as quickly as possible. However, you should choose the items of your literary diet as carefully as those of your nutritional diet or you will suffer from mental indigestion! In other words, *don't over-read*.

BILLING, D. H. M. (1976) *Practical Procedures for Nurses*, 13th ed. London: Baillière Tindall.

CAPE, B. F. AND DOBSON, P. (1974) *Baillière's Nurses' Dictionary*, 18th ed. London: Baillière Tindall.

HECTOR, W. (1976) *Modern Nursing. Theory and Practice*, 6th ed. London: Heinemann Medical.

HOUGHTON, M. AND JEE, L. A. (1971) *Baillière's Pocketbook of Ward Information*, 12th ed. London: Baillière Tindall.

HULL, E. J. AND ISAACS, B. J. (1976) *Quizzes and Questions for Nurses. Book A: Medical Nursing and Paediatric Nursing. Book B: Surgical Nursing and Geriatric Nursing*. London: Baillière Tindall.

MOUNTJOY, P. AND WYTHE, B. (1970) *Nursing Care of the Unconscious Patient*. London: Baillière Tindall.

PEARCE, E. C. (1975) *General Textbook of Nursing*, 19th ed. London: Faber & Faber.

SMITH, D. W. et al. (1971) *Care of the Adult Patient*, 3rd ed. New York: Lippincott. (Very useful for its case studies.)

For detailed study of topics at a more advanced level, consult the Nurses' Aids Series, published by Baillière Tindall.

Journals
Nursing Times and *Nursing Mirror* are weekly journals for the profession. They contain articles covering all aspects of nursing, the authors being nurses, doctors and technicians.

Both journals also provide news of events and people, book reviews and correspondence columns. They are a useful source of information for project work.

INDEX

abortion, 186
absorption, 126
accidents in the home, 24–7
    general prevention, 24
acetabulum, 135, 136
acne, 197
acute confusional states, 36–7
acute nephritis, 177–8
acute rheumatism, 145
Addison's disease, 227
adhesive dressings, 88–9
admission of patients to hospital,
    51–4, 109–10, 213
adolescence, 2–3
adolescent patients, 112
adrenaline, 227
adrenals, 226–7
adrenocorticotrophic hormone, 225
adulthood, 3
aged see the elderly
aggression in psychiatric patients,
    47–8
alimentary tract, 151–3
allergic reactions to drugs, 75–6
amenorrhoea, 185
amylases, 153, 154
anaemia, 160
anatomy and physiology of the
    systems see under each system
androgens, 228
angina pectoris, 165
ankle, 145
anorexia nervosa, 39–40
antibiotics, 94, 166–7
antibodies, 95, 158
anticoagulants, 166
antidepressants, 42–3
antidiuretic hormone, 226

antifungal agents, 94
antigens, 95, 158
antiseptics, 102
anus, 153
anxiety states, 38–40
apex beat, measurement of, 69–70
arachnid parasites, 22
arm,
    bones, 134–5
    joints, 144–5
    muscles, 141
arteries, 162, 163
arteriosclerosis, 163
arthritis, 145
artificial respiration, 84–5
atherosclerosis, 163
atmospheric pollution, 12
autoclaving, 102
autonomic nervous system, 202,
    205–6

babies,
    bathing, 106–7
    clothing, 106
    exercise, 106
    feeding, 107–8
    health supervision, 108–9
    normal development, 1–2, 105–6
    nursing see paediatric patients
babyhood, 1–2, 105–6
bacilli, 93
backrests, 58
bacteria, 93, 94
bactericides, 102
bacteriostats, 102
balance, 222

bandages, 87–9
barrier nursing, 99–101
bathing of patients, 192–4
bed bathing, 193–4
bed bugs, 21–2
bed cradles, 58
bed linen, contaminated, handling of, 57
bed-making, 55–7
bed patients,
    aids to comfort, 57–8, 149
    lifting, 62
    nursing positions, 58–62, 149
bed sores see pressure areas and sores
bed-wetting, 177
behaviour therapy, 44–5
behavioural disorders, 35–42, 124
benign growths, 123
beta-blocking, 166
biceps, 141
bile, 153
birth control clinic nurses, 33
bladder see gall bladder; urinary bladder
blanket baths, 193–4
bleeding see haemorrhage
blood,
    disorders, 160–1
    kidneys and, 170–1
    physiology, 157–9
    see also cardiovascular system; haemorrhage
blood cells,
    manufacture, 128–30
    types, 157–8
blood clots, 163, 165
blood groups, 158–9
blood pressure,
    high, reduction of, 166
    measurement, 70
blood transfusion, 158–60
body lice, 21
boiling for sterilization, 101–2
bones,
    anatomy and physiology, 128–38
    diseases, 138
    fractures, 130, 138–40
    in principal joints, 144–5

bowel movements,
    breathless patients and, 149
    elderly patients and, 116–17
    normal, maintenance of, 8
brain, 202–5
    tumours, 208
brain stem, 203, 204
breastbone, 131
breathlessness see dyspnoea
broad slings, 91
burns and scalds, first aid for, 200–1
bursitis, 145

caecum, 153
Caesarian section, 181
calcium, 15
calories, 17–18
cancers see neoplasms
capillaries, 162–3
carbohydrates,
    bodily storage, 18
    calorific value, 18
    enzymes and, 153, 154
    functions, 13
    in milk, 16
    sources, 13
cardiac arrest, 84, 85–6
cardiac disease see heart, disease of
cardiac massage, external, 85–6
cardiovascular system,
    anatomy and physiology of, 161–3
    disorders, 163–7
    see also entries beginning 'blood'
carpals, 134–5, 145
carriers, of infection, 97
cartilaginous joints, 143
cataract, 220
catheterization of the urinary bladder, 176
cells, 120–1
    see also blood cells; nerve tissue
central nervous system, 202–5
central sterile supply departments, 102
cerebellum, 203, 204
cerebral palsy, 209
cerebral tumours, 208

cerebrospinal fluid, 203, 204
  lumbar puncture and, 211–12
cerebrovascular accident, 163, 207
cerebrum, 203, 204
cervical smear, 180
chemical sterilization, 102
chemicals, household, accidents involving, 27
chest bones, 131
Cheyne–Stokes breathing, 69
chilblains, 7
childhood, 2
children,
  accidents at home, 24, 27
  crying, significance of types of, 111
  nursing of, see paediatric patients
    see also babies
choroid, 215–16
chromosomes, 121
chronic renal failure, 178
circulatory system see cardiovascular system
clavicle, 134–5
clean air, 12
clinical thermometers, 63
clitoris, 182–3
cocci, 93
coccyx, 133, 135
coitus, 179
collar-and-cuff slings, 92
collar bone, 134–5
college nurses, 33
colon, 153
colostomy, 155–6
commensals, 93
communal health, 10–12
communicating with patients see nurse–patient communication
community nurses, 29–32
community psychiatric nurses, 32, 50
conception, 179
confabulation, 37
confusional states, 36–7
congenital disorders, definition of, 123
conjunctiva, 216
  specimen-collecting of, 219

consent forms for surgery, 79
Control of Infection Officers, 97
Controlled Drugs, 72, 73
corns, 7
coronary arteries, 164, 165
coronary attack, 165
corticoids, 227
cradles, bed, 58
cranial nerves, 205
cranium, 130
crêpe bandages, 88
cretinism, 226
cross-infection, 97–8, 192
crying in children, significance of types of, 111
Cushing's syndrome, 227
cyanosis, 164
cystitis, 178
cystocele, 181
cytology, 120–1 see also blood cells; nerve tissue
cytoplasm, 120

day hospitals, 119
deaf patients, 222–3
degenerative disorders, definition of, 123
deltoid, 142
delusions,
  definition of, 36
  management of patients with, 48
dementia, 37
depression, 37–8 see also manic depressive psychosis
dermatitis, 197
dermatology see skin
dermis, 187–8
desensitization in treatment of phobic anxiety, 45
detergents, 102
diabetes mellitus, 228, 228–9
  diet for, 19
diaphragm, 142
diarrhoea, 155
diets, 18–19
  in nephritis, 177–8

diets (*continued*)
  preoperative, 79, 110
diffusion, 126, 170
digestive system,
  accessory organs, 155
  alimentary tract, 151–3
  anatomy and physiology, 151–5
  enzymes, 152, 153–4
  faeces and, 155
  operations, 155–6
  sphincters, 153, 154
dilatation and curettage, 180
diseases and disorders,
  classification, 123
  see also individual conditions and
    systems
disinfectants, 102
dissolution, 125–6
District nurses, 29–32
diuretics, 166
dorsal position, 59
drug trolleys, 72
drugs,
  abuse of, 42
  administration, 73–8
    by injection, 76–8
    by mouth, 75–6
  in treatment of,
    heart disease, 165–7
    infections, 94
    mental illness, 42–3
    ophthalmic conditions, 218
    skin conditions, 198–9, 200
  measurement of, 73–4
  preoperative, 79, 80
dry heat for sterilization, 102
duodenum, 152
dysmenorrhoea, 185
dyspnoea, 69, 149–50, 164

ear,
  anatomy and physiology, 221–2
  disorders, 222
  syringing, 222
ears, discharge from in unconscious-
    ness, 214
eczema, 197

elbow, 135, 145
elderly, the, 3–4, 113–14
  accidents at home, 24
  illnesses and care of *see* geriatric
    patients
electric blankets and pads, 58
electrical accidents in the home, 24–5
electroconvulsive therapy, 43–4
embolism, 163
embryos, development of, 121
emergencies in the ward, 84–6
endemic outbreaks of infectious
    diseases, 97
endocarditis, 165
endocardium, 164
endocrine system, 224–9
  anatomy and physiology, 225–8
  disorders, 123, 226, 227, 228–9
endometrium, 184
enuresis, 177
enzymes, 152, 153–4
epidemics, 97
epidermis, 187–8
epilepsy, 207–8
erythrocytes, 157, 169
erythropoietin, 228
exercise, bodily, 6
  of the elderly in hospital, 114,
    115–16, 117
expiration, pulmonary, 148
extensors, digital, 142
eye,
  anatomy and physiology, 142,
    215–17
  disorders, 220
eye drops and irrigation, 218–19
eyelashes, cutting of, 219
eyes, care of in unconsciousness, 213

face muscles, 142
faeces,
  significance of types of in children,
    111
  specimen-collection, 155
  see also bowel movements
Fallopian tubes, 183
family planning clinic nurses, 33

fats,
   bodily storage, 18
   calorific value, 18
   enzymes and, 153, 154
   functions, 13–14
   in milk, 16
   sources, 13–14
feeding,
   babies, 107–8
   breathless patient, 149
   geriatric patients, 116, 117
   other than by mouth, 13
   psychiatric patients, 48
   unconscious patients, 214
   see also diets; food
feet, care of, 7, 136
   in elderly patients, 116
   see also foot
female reproductive system,
   abortion, 186
   anatomy and physiology, 182–5
   conception, 179
   see also gynaecology
femur, 135–6, 145
feverish patients,
   nursing, 102–4
   tepid sponging, 66–8
fibrositis, 143
fibrous joints, 143
fibula, 136, 137, 145
filtration, 127, 173
first aid,
   burns and scalds, 200–1
   fractures, 139
fission, cellular, 120–1
flat feet, 7, 136
fleas, 21, 97
flexors, digital, 142
flies (houseflies), 20
fluoridation of water, 11
follicle-stimulating hormone, 225
food,
   bowel action, 8, 111
   constituents, 13–16, 170
   contamination, 17, 20, 22–3, 96–7
   digestion, 151–4
   function, 13–16, 17–18
   hormonal role in metabolism, 224–8

food, (continued)
   inadequate intake by the elderly,
      113–14
   poisoning, 17, 96–7
   water constituent of, 170
   see also anorexia nervosa; diets;
      feeding
foot, bones and arches, 136–8
   care, 7, 136
   elderly patients, 116
fore-brain, 203, 204
fractures of bones, 130, 138
   treatment for, 139–40
frequency of urine, 177
functional disorders, definition, 35–6
fungi, 23, 93, 94

gall bladder, 153
gametes, 121
gamma-ray irradiation, 102
garages, household, accidents in, 27
gardens, household, accidents in, 27
gas, household, accidents, 25, 223
gases, physics of, 125
gastro-intestinal tract see alimentary
   tract
gastrocnemius, 142
gastrostomy, 13
genital systems see female reproductive system; male reproductive
   system
geriatric patients,
   common diseases, 114–115
   day hospitals, 119
   hospital care, 115–19
      bowel attention, 116–17
      discharge, 118
      feeding, 116
      mobility, 115–16
      recreation, 117–18
      visitors, 118
German measles see rubella
glaucoma, 220
glucocorticoids, 227
gluten-free diets, 19
gluteus maximus, 142
glycogen, 153, 227

goitre, 16, 226
gonads *see* ovaries; testes
grand mal, 207
growth hormone, 225
gynaecology, 179–81
    abortion, 186
    operations, 180–1
    procedures, 180
haematology *see entries beginning
    blood*
haemoglobin, 157
haemophilia, 161
haemoptysis, 86, 164
haemorrhage, 82, 84, 167, 185
haemorrhoids, 163
hair,
    nurses', care of, 8
    patients', care of, 194
hallucinations,
    definition of, 36
    management of patients with, 48
hamstrings, 142
hand,
    bones, 134–5
    muscles, 142
head lice, 21
health,
    personal, 5–9
    public, 10–12
health visitors, 28–9, 109
hearing *see* ear
heart,
    anatomy and physiology, 161–2,
        164
    apex beat, 69–70
    disease, of
        drugs used, 165–7
        nursing, 164
        sites, 164
        symptoms, 164
        types, 165
    see also cardiac arrest
heart rate, drugs affecting, 166
heat,
    bodily regulation of, 189–91
    dry, for sterilization, 102
    see also temperature
heat stroke, 191

helminths, 22–3
hemiplegia, definition of, 209
herpes zoster, 197
high-calorie diets, 18
high-protein diets, 18–19
hind-brain, 203, 204
hip, 135, 136, 145
histology,
    blood, 157–9
    bones, 128–30
    nephrons, 173
    nerve tissue, 206
    skin, 187–8
    see also cells
home,
    accidents, 24–7
    care of, 9
    pests and parasites, 20–3
hormones, 224–9
hostility in psychiatric patients, 47–8
hot water-bottles, 57–8
houseflies, 20
'housemaids' knee', 145
housing, 11–12
human life-span, 1–4
human skeleton, 129
humerus, 134–5, 144, 145
hydrochloric acid, 152
hydrocortisone, 227
hygiene,
    cow's milk, 16, 96
    food, 17, 20, 22–3, 96–7
    oral, 48, 103, 149, 213
    personal *see* personal health and
        hygiene
    pests and parasites and, 20–3, 97
    wards, 98
    water , 22–3, 96
    see also infection, transmission of
hymen, 183
hyperglycaemia, 228–9
hyperpyrexia, 66
    see also pyrexia
hypersensitivity to drugs, 76
hypertension, 166
hypnotics, 43
hypodermic injections, 77
hypoglycaemia, 228–9

hypotensive drugs, 166
hypothermia, 66
hysterectomy, 180–1
hysteria, 39

ileostomy, 156
ileum, 152–3
ilium, 135, 136
immunity, 95–6
impetigo, 197
incontinence,
    nursing care, 195, 196
    urinary, 177
industrial therapy in mental illness,
    44
infantile paralysis, 208
infants see babies; children; paedi-
    atric patients,
infection,
    immunity, 95–6
    inflammation, 94–5
    micro-organisms causing, 93
    transmission, 96–8
        prevention, 98–102
    treatment, 94
    see also hygiene
infectious diseases,
    definition, 123
    notifiable, 99
    types of outbreak, 97
inflammation, 94–5
ingrowing toenails, 7
injections, techniques, 76–8
innocent growths, 123
innominate bones, 135, 136, 145
insect parasites and pests, 20–2
insight, psychiatric, definition, 36
insomnia, 5–6, 48–9
inspiration, pulmonary, 148
insulin, 19, 153, 228, 229
intermenstrual bleeding, 185
intervertebral discs, 133
intestines, small and large, 152–3
intramuscular injections, 77–8, 142
intravenous feeding, 13
intravenous injections, 78
involuntary muscles, 142–3

involvement of nurses with psy-
    chiatric patients, 47
iodine, 16, 226
iron, 15
irrigation of the eye, 218–19
ischaemic heart disease, 165
ischium, 135, 136
islets of Langerhans, 228
itch-mites, 22

jejunum, 152
joints, 143–5

kaolin poultices, 197–8
kidneys, 170–2, 173, 177–8, 228
kilojoules, 17–18
'kiss of life', 84–5
kitchens, accidents in, 25–6
knee, 136, 145

labia majora and minora, 182
lacrimal glands, 216
lactogenic hormone, 225
large intestine, 153
larynx, 147
Lawson–Tait cardiac bed, 60
Lawson–Tait–Fowler bed, 60
left lateral position, 61
left-sided heart failure, 165
leucocytes, 95, 157–8, 169
leukaemia, 160
lice, 21
life-span, human, 1–4
lifting of patients, 62
liniments, 198
linen, bed, contaminated, handling
    of, 57
lipases, 153, 154
liquids, physics of, 125
liver, 153
lotions, 199
low-fat diets, 19
low-protein diets, 19
low-salt diets, 19
lower limb,
    bones, 135–8

lower limb, (*continued*)
joints, 145
muscles, 142
lumbar puncture, 211–12
lungs, 148
luteinizing hormone, 225
lymphatic system, 168–9
lymphocytes, 169

male reproductive system,
anatomy and physiology of, 181–2
conception and, 179
malignant growths, 123–4
manic-depressive psychosis, 41
mastoiditis, 222
medicines *see* drugs
medulla oblongata, 204–5
meiosis, 121
melaena stools, 155
melanin, 187, 188
meninges, 203
meningitis, 208
menorrhagia, 185
menstrual cycle, 184–5
menstruation and personal hygiene, 8
Mental Health Services Act 1959, 34, 35
mental illness *see* psychiatric disease
metacarpals, 134–5
metatarsals, 136, 137
micro-organisms, 93
see also infection
micturition, 172
disorders, 176–7
mid-brain, 204
middle-age, 3
midstream specimen of urine, 175
midwifery, definition, 180
milk, 16–17, 96, 107–8
mineral salts,
calorific value, 18
functions, 15–16
in milk, 16
sources, 15–16
mineralocorticoids, 227
miotics, definition, 218
mites, 22
mitosis, 121

mobility of the elderly patient, 114, 115–16, 117
molecules, 125
monoplegia, definition, 209
mons veneris, 182
mosquitoes, 20–1
mouth,
care of, 48, 103, 149, 213
digestive function of, 151
mouth-to-mouth respiration, 84–5
multiple sclerosis, 209
muscles,
anatomy and physiology, 5, 141–3
diseases, 143
muscular dystrophy, 143
myasthenia gravis, 143
mydriatics, definition of, 218
myocardium, 164
myxoedema, 226

neoplasms, 123–4, 208
nephritis, 177–8
nephron, 172, 173
nerve tissue, 206
nervous system,
anatomy and physiology, 202–7
autonomic system, 202, 205–6
central system, 202–5
disorders of, 207–9
nursing, 210–14
nerve tissue, 206
peripheral nerves of, 205
reflex arc of, 206–7
nettle rash, 197
neurology *see* nervous system
neurones, 206
neurosis, definition, 36
noradrenaline, 227
nose, 146–7, 223
notifiable infectious diseases, 99
nuclei, cellular, 120–1
nurse–patient communication, involving
children, 109, 110
elderly patients, 115, 118
patients in general, 51–2
psychiatric patients, 46–7

nurses in the community, 28–33, 50,
    108–9
nutrition *see* food

obesity, 18
obstetrics, definition, 179
occupational health nurses, 32–3
occupational health service for hos-
    pital staff, 8–9
occupational therapy, in,
    geriatric illness, 117
    mental illness, 44
oedema, 164
oesophagus, 151
oestrogen, 228
oil heaters and lamps, accidents
    involving, 26
ointments, 199
old age, 3–4, 113–14
    see also elderly, the; geriatric
        patients
ophthalmia neonatorum, 220
ophthalmology *see* eye
ophthalmoplegia, definition, 209
oral hygiene, 48, 103, 149, 213
organic psychiatric disorders, defi-
    nition, 35
organs, definition, 121
orthopnoeic position, 60
osmosis, 126–7, 170
osseous system *see* bones
osteoarthritis, 145
osteomalacia, 138
osteomyelitis, 138
otitis media, 222
ova, 121, 179, 183, 184
ovaries, 181, 183, 228
oxygen, 167
oxytocin, 226

paediatric patients,
    home nursing, 109
    hospital admission, 109–10
    observations, 110–11

paediatric patients, (*continued*)
    visiting of, 111–12
    ward routine, 112
    see also babies
paediatrics, definition, 179
Paget's disease, 138
palpitations, 164
pancreas, 153, 228
paraffin heaters and lamps, accidents
    involving, 26
paralysis agitans, 208–9
paraplegia, definition, 209
parasites, 20–3, 97
parasympathetic nerves, 205, 206
parathormone, 227
parathyroids, 227
paresis, definition, 209
paints, 198
Parkinson's disease, 208–9
patella, 145
pediculosis, 21
pelvis bones, 135, 136
penis, 181
pepsin, 152
pepsinogen, 152
pericarditis, 165
pericardium, 164
perineum, 183
periods, monthly, 8, 184–5
peripheral nerves, 205
peristalsis, 151
personal health and hygiene,
    food, 17, 96–7
    for nurses, 5–9, 96, 98, 191–2
    pests and parasites, 20–3
personality behaviour disorders, 41–
    42
pests, 20, 22, 97
petit mal, 207
phagocytes, 95
phalanges, 134–5, 136, 137
pharynx, 147, 151
phobias, 38
    behaviour therapy, 44–5
phosphorus, 15
physical principles, 125–7
physiology *see under each system*
piles, 163

pineal gland, 228
pituitary gland, 225–6
plasma, blood, 157
plaster of Paris appliances, 89–91, 139–40
platelets, blood, 157, 158
plegia, definition, 209
poliomyelitis, 208
polycythaemia, 161
pons, 204
postoperative care, 81–2, 111
    complications, 82–3
posture, bodily, 6
poultices, 197–8
premedication, 80
preoperative preparation, 79–81, 110
prescriptions, 73, 74, 75
presenile dementia, 37
pressure areas and sores, 194–7, 213
progesterone, 228
prolapse of uterus, 181
prolapsed intervertebral disc, 133
prostate, 181
proteases, 154
proteins,
    bodily storage, 18
    calorific value, 18
    enzymes and, 152, 154
    functions, 13
    in milk, 16
    sources of, 13
    special diets, 18–19
psoriasis, 197
psychiatric disease,
    attitudes and treatment, 34–5, 49–50
    nursing see psychiatric nursing
    terminological definitions, 35–6, 124
    treatment, 42–5
    varieties, 36–42
psychiatric nursing, 45–9, 50
    aggression and hostility, 47–8
    feeding in, 48
    in the community, 50
    involvement with patients, 47
    sleep, 48–9
    suicide, 49

psychiatric nursing, (*continued*)
    verbal communication, 46–7, 48
psychopathy, 42
psychosis, 36, 41
psychotherapy, 42
pubis, 135, 136
public health, 10–12
public health nurses, 29
pulleys, bed, 58
pulmonary system see respiration
pulse,
    drugs affecting, 166
    measurement of, 68–9, 110–11
    radial, 135
pyelonephritis, 178
pyrexia, 66, 191
    nursing of patients, 102–4
    tepid sponging, 66–8

quadriceps, 142
quadriplegia, definition, 209

radium, gynaecological use, 180
radius, 134–5, 145
rats, 22, 97
records, patients', maintenance of, 70–1
rectal thermometers, 63, 65
rectocele, 181
rectum, 153
recumbent position, 58
red blood cells, 157, 169
reflex arc, 206
refuse collection, 11
renal failure, 178
    for renal matters in general see kidneys
rennin, 152
report-writing, 70–1
reproductive systems see female reproductive system; male reproductive system
respiration,
    anatomy and physiology, 146–8

respiration, (*continued*)
  difficulty, 149
    nursing, for, 149–50
  failure of, 82, 84–5
rest, bodily, 5
retention of urine, 176
retina, 216
reverse barrier nursing, 100–1
rhesus factor, 159
rheumatic fever, 145
rheumatoid arthritis, 145
ribs, 131
rickets, 138
right-sided heart failure, 165
rigor, 66–7
ringworm, 23, 93
roundworms, 23
rubber rings, 58
rubella, immunisation of girls, 95–6, 99

sacral rings, 58
sacrum, 133, 135
St John's slings, 91–2
salpingo-oophorectomy with hysterectomy, 181
scabies, 22
scalds, *see* burns and scalds
scapula, 134–5, 144
Schedule 1 Poisons, 72–3
schizophrenias, 40–1
school nurses, 37
sclera, 215
scorpions, 22
sebaceous glands, 188
sedatives, 43
semi-prone position, 60–1
semi-recumbent position, 58
seminal vesicles, 181
sense organs,
  ear, 221–3
  eye, 215–20
  nose, 223
  tongue, 223
sewage disposal, 11
sex corticoids, 227
sexual deviations, 41–2

sexual intercourse, 179
shingles, 197
shock, 82
shoulder, 134–5, 144
Sims's position, 62
skeletal system *see* bones
skeleton, human, 129
skin,
  anatomy and physiology, 187–8
  disorders, 197
    nursing and treatment, 197–200
  functions, 188–9
  heat regulation, 189–91
  nurses', care of, 191
skull, 130–1
  muscles of, 142
sleep, 5–6, 48–9
slings, 91–2
'slipped disc', 133
small intestine, 152–3
smell, sense of, 223
sodium, 15, 19
solids, physics of, 125
sound, 221–2
special senses *see* sense organs
specific gravity, 174
sperms, 121, 179
sphincters, 153, 154, 172
spiders, 22
spinal column, 131–3
  cord, 202–3, 205
  nerves, 205
spirilla, 93
spleen, 169
splints, 89–91
sponging, 66–8
sporadic outbreaks of infectious diseases, 97
squint, 220
starch poultices, 198
steam bathing of the eye, 220
steam sterilization, 102
sterilization and cleaning, 101–2
  of babies' bottles, 108
sternum, 131
stoma, 155
stomach, 152
stools *see* faeces

strabismus, 220
stroke, 163, 207
subacute nephritis, 178
subcutaneous injections, 77
subnormal temperature, 66
suicide, 49
sun stroke, 191
suppression of urine, 177
suprarenals, 226–7
surgical patients,
    postoperative care, 81–3, 111
    preoperative care, 79–81, 110
sweat glands, 188
sympathetic nerves, 205–6
syncope, 164
synovial joints, 143–4
syringing the ear, 222
systems, anatomical, classification of,
    122

talking and listening to patients *see*
    nurse–patient communication
talus, 145
tapeworms, 23
tarsals, 136, 137
taste, 223
temperature,
    bodily regulation, 189–91
    of wards, 63
    patients',
        abnormal, types, 66
        taking, 63, 64–6, 110–11
    scales of, 63–4
tepid sponging, 66–8
testes, 181, 228
testosterone, 228
thermometers, 63
    see also temperature
thorax, bones of, 131
thought-blocking, 41
thousand-calorie diets, 18
threadworms, 22–3
thrombus, 165
thymus, 228
thyroid, 16, 226, 228–9
thyroid-stimulating hormone, 225

thyrotoxicosis, 226
thyroxine, 226
tibia, 136, 137, 145
ticks, 22
tinea, 23
tongue, 223
tonsils and tonsillitis, 169
trachea, 147
tracheostomy, 150
tranquillizers, 43
transfusion, blood, 158–60
trauma, definition, 124
triangular bandages, 88, 91–2
triceps, 141
trunk, areas, 188, 189
trypsin, 153
tumours, neoplastic *see* neoplasms

ulna, 134–5, 145
unconscious patients, nursing, 212–
    214
    postoperative, 81–2
universal thermometers, 63
upper limb,
    bones, 134–5
    joints, 144–5
    muscles, 141
upright position in bed, 60
uraemia, 178
ureters, 172
urinary bladder, 172, 178, 214
    catheterization, 176
urinary system,
    anatomy and physiology, 170–3
    disorders of, 176–8
urine,
    appearance, 174
    catheterization, 176
    composition, 173
    incontinence, 177
    production, 173
    retention, 176
    specimen-collection, 175
    testing of, 174
        storage of reagents, 73
urology *see* urinary system; urine

urticaria, 197
uterus, 180–1, 183–4

vaccination, 95–6
vagina, 183
  douching, 180
varicose veins, 163
vas deferens, 181
vasoconstrictors, 166
vasodilators, 166
vasopressin, 226
veins, 163
venereal diseases, 185–6
vertebrae, 131–3
villi, 153
viruses, 93, 94
vision *see* eye
visiting hospital,
  breathless patients, 150
  children, 111–12

visiting hospital, (*continued*)
  the elderly, 118
vitamins,
  calorific value of, 18
  functions of, 14–15
  in milk, 16
  sources, 14–15
voluntary muscles, 141–2
vomiting, postanaesthetic, 82–3
vulva, 182

ward emergencies, 84–6
washing patients, 192
water,
  bodily function, 170–1
  contamination, 22–3, 96
  public supply, 10–11
white blood cells, 95, 157–8, 169
worms, parasitic, 22–3, 155
wrist, 134–5, 145